Understanding Leukemias, Lymphomas and Myelomas

Tariq I Mughal
Professor of Medicine and Hematology/Oncology
University of Massachusetts Medical School
Worcester, Massachusetts, USA

John M Goldman
Fogarty Scholar and Professor of Leukemia Biology
Hematology Branch
National Heart, Lung and Blood Institute
Bethesda, Maryland, USA

Sabena T Mughal
Medical Student
Imperial College London
London, UK

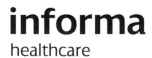
informa
healthcare

© 2006 Taylor & Francis, an imprint of the Taylor & Francis Group

First published in the United Kingdom in 2006
by Taylor & Francis, an imprint of the Taylor & Francis Group, 2 Park Square, Milton
Park, Abingdon, Oxon OX14 4RN

Tel.:   +44 (0) 20 7017 6000
Fax.:   +44 (0) 20 7017 6699
E-mail.:   info.medicine@tandf.co.uk
Website: http://www.tandf.co.uk/medicine

Second printing 2007

Although every effort has been made to ensure that all owners of copyright material
have been acknowledged in this publication, we would be glad to acknowledge in
subsequent reprints or editions any omissions brought to our attention.

Although every effort has been made to ensure that drug doses and other information
are presented accurately in this publication, the ultimate responsibility rests with the
prescribing physician. Neither the publishers nor the authors can be held responsible
for errors or for any consequences arising from the use of information contained herein.
For detailed prescribing information or instructions on the use of any product or
procedure discussed herein, please consult the prescribing information or instructional
material issued by the manufacturer.

A CIP record for this book is available from the British Library.

Library of Congress Cataloging-in-Publication Data

Data available on application

ISBN 1-84184-409-8
ISBN 978-1-84184-409-1

Distributed in North and South America by
Taylor & Francis
2000 NW Corporate Blvd
Boca Raton, FL 33431, USA
Within Continental USA
Tel: 800 272 7737; Fax: 800 374 3401
Outside Continental USA
Tel: 561 994 0555; Fax: 561 361 6018
E-mail: orders@crcpress.com

Distributed in the rest of the world by
Thomson Publishing Services
Cheriton House
North Way
Andover, Hampshire SP10 5BE, UK
Tel.:   44 (0)1264 332424
E-mail: salesorder.tandf@thomsonpublishingservices.co.uk

Composition by J&L Composition, Filey, North Yorkshire

Printed and bound in India by Replika Press Pvt. Ltd

Dedication

This book is dedicated to our patients with blood cancers, past and present, who by motivating and encouraging us, made this work possible. Sadly many have now died, but we hope that the information collated will be of benefit to the patients of the future, their relatives and their healthcare team. TM also dedicates it to the memory of his dear late father, who was always a source of enormous strength, guidance and love.

Know then thyself, presume not God to scan;
The proper study of mankind is man.
Placed on this isthmus of a middle state,
A being darkly wise, and rudely great:
With too much knowledge for the sceptic side,
With too much weakness for the stoic's pride,
He hangs between; in doubt to act or rest,
In doubt to deem himself a god, or beast;
In doubt his mind or body to prefer,
Born but to die, and reas'ning but to err;
Alike in ignorance, his reason such,
Whether he thinks too little, or too much.

Alexander Pope, *An Essay on Man* Epistle 2 (1733) 1.1
see Charron 192:2

Contents

Notes on the authors

Tariq I Mughal is a Professor of Medicine and Hematology/Oncology at the University of Massachusetts Medical School, Worcester, Massachusetts, USA specializing in hematologic cancers. He is also a Consultant Hematologist at the Dartford and Guy's and St. Thomas's Hospitals, London, UK and a Visiting Professor at the European School of Oncology, Bellinzona, Switzerland. He graduated from St. George's Hospital Medical School, London, UK, and received his postgraduate training at the Westminister Hospital Medical School Hospitals, London, the University of Colorado School of Medicine, Denver, Colorado, USA and the Hammersmith Hospital and the Royal Postgraduate Medical School, London, UK.

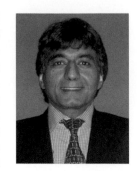

John M Goldman is a Fogarty Scholar at the National Heart, Lung and Blood Institute, National Institutes of Health, Bethesda, Maryland, USA, specializing in leukemias. He is also a Professor of Leukemia Biology and a Consultant Hematologist at the Hammersmith Hospital at Imperial College School of Medicine, London, UK. He graduated from the University of Oxford, UK and received his postgraduate training at the Massachusetts General Hospital, Boston, USA; the University of Miami, Florida, USA and the Hammersmith Hospital and the Royal Postgraduate Medical School, London, UK.

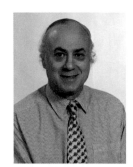

Sabena T Mughal is a medical student at the Imperial College London, London, UK. She attended Withington Girls' School, Manchester, UK and carried out pre-medical elective studies at the University of Colorado Health Sciences Center, Denver, Colorado, USA. She is involved in a number of charitable and voluntary projects in various medical fields, in addition to composing music.

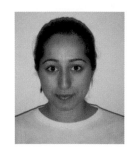

Foreword by José Carreras

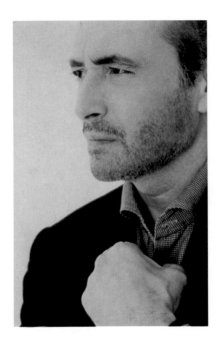

President, International José Carreras Foundation, Barcelona, Spain

Some years ago I was kindly invited by Dr. Mughal and Dr. Goldman to write the foreword of a previous work of theirs. Now, together with Dr. Mughal Jr., they give me the opportunity to praise their talent and dedication again and I am very pleased to do it.

The authors of this book devote time and energy to the advancement of science and to the care of patients. But if this was not a big enough contribution, they are also concerned about helping the patients and their families confront the harsh reality of the disease from an integral perspective. Such perspective stresses the fact that the patient and the family are human beings with more than just a physiological dimension.

It has been repeatedly published and advised that a hopeful attitude from the patient and the strong support of the family are crucial elements in the treatment process. I am not of course prepared to explain why this is so. However I can confirm that, at least in my case, despite logical moments of weakness and doubt, any positive word, thought or wish was fundamental for a successful recovery. The patient must believe that, in addition to science and professional excellence, his or her soul plays a decisive role.

In many aspects of life, we cannot be determined, enthusiastic or courageous if we do not understand what is happening around us. Drs. Mughal and Dr. Goldman help patients and families make this first necessary step in a situation where fear and uncertainty can be balanced by knowledge, information and correct expectations.

Finally, let me share with you what I recall as being the fundamental source of strength in my recovery; even if there is only a small chance of survival, that particular chance is yours and the one you fight for.

Foreword by James O Armitage, MD

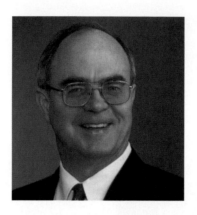

Joe Shapiro Professor of Internal Medicine, University of Nebraska Medical Center, Omaha, and Dean, Nebraska School of Medicine, Omaha, Nebraska, USA; ex-President of the American Society of Clinical Oncology and ex-President of the American Society for Blood and Marrow Transplant Research

The relationship of physicians and their patients has changed dramatically over the last few decades. Previously, young physicians were often taught to keep an 'emotional distance' between themselves and their patients in order to allow objective decision making. Today, increasingly, and perhaps particularly in hematology and oncology, physicians and patients have become friends. It was once expected that patients would accept a physician's instructions promptly and without debate – in fact physicians would sometimes become angry if a patient questioned their opinion and advice. Today, particularly in the United States, informed patients who take it upon themselves to be active participants in their own care are increasingly common. This is partly a reflection of the increasing amount of information available to patients that allows them to be partners in making informed decisions. Often obtained via the Internet, the information patients find can be of high quality but, unfortunately, sometimes can be inaccurate, misleading and harmful. This book is an excellent and important example of useful and accurate information – particularly for patients who suffer from hematologic malignancies.

I have always felt that informed patients should make strategic decisions about their care. Here I am using strategic in a military sense, as opposed to tactics. Making the decision about the overall approach to their illness (e.g. taking risks in an attempt to cure a disease while minimizing risks and avoiding unpleasant treatments if at all possible) should be in the province of an informed patient – at least if they wish to make these decisions. However, I counsel patients that once they have given an overall direction for their care it is wise to take the physician's advice on tactics (e.g. the specific chemotherapy regimen, the specific antibiotic). This presumes that the patient has found a physician with whom they can communicate, who they believe is knowledgeable and whom they trust.

Perhaps in days past, when very little was known about mechanisms of disease, it was wise that patients didn't realize how poorly informed their physicians actually were. However, and particularly in the field of hematologic malignancies, new insights into these disorders have dramatically improved our ability to treat effectively. There are almost no situations where management cannot be approached hopefully, and many situations where our treatments might effect cure. Knowing the state of affairs today is likely to encourage rather than discourage patients. A book such as this, written in language that can be readily understood by patients and their families, provides an invaluable asset for those who want to be informed. The information is consistently presented in a hopeful, clear and honest way. It takes the same information that could be found in a textbook of hematologic oncology or in *New England Journal of Medicine* reviews and translates the information into a more understandable language.

This is a book that physicians who want patients as 'partners' in their care should recommend. Reading these chapters will alleviate the anxiety of the unknown for many patients while leaving them with a sense of hope that is appropriate for the care of the disorders. It not only offers an excellent overview for patients, but could be utilized by physicians and nurses in training and other medical professionals to their great benefit.

A strength of this book is, certainly, the senior authors. They have extensive experience in the management of patients with hematologic malignancies. They have made important contributions to our understanding of the biology of leukemia and the treatment of patients with these disorders. Together with their junior author, they have managed to make this book positive throughout and full of energy. They clearly want patients to look forward and face the future positively.

Acknowledgments

We thank our many colleagues, patients and friends for reading the various drafts and for diligently discussing the contents and apologize that they are not named individually. We thank our Greek friends for their help with the translations; Professor Barbara Bain for providing some of the figures; and Robert Peden of Taylor and Francis for his professionalism and patience, particularly with the endless deadlines! TM and SM should like to thank his mother/her grandmother (respectively) for loving support. SM is responsible for the cover design.

Publisher's acknowledgments

The Publishers wish to acknowledge gratefully the following, who have kindly allowed their figures to be used in this publication.

Armitage O, Cavalli F, Zucca E, Longo D. *Text Atlas of Lymphomas (revised edition)*; Martin Dunitz: London 2002, for Figure 4.27

Beale R for Figure 11.1

Blood for Figures 8.4, 9.9, 9.11, 9.13

Gorczyca W, Weisberger J, Emmons FN. *Atlas of Differential Diagnosis in Neoplastic Hematopathology*; Taylor and Francis: Abingdon 2004, for Figures 3.10, 3.11, 4.17, 4.22, 4.31, 4.32 and 5.16

Hoffbrand V, Pettit JE. *Essential Haematology (third edition)* Blackwell: Oxford 1993, for Figures 2.9, 3.8, 5.15, 5.22

Mufti GJ, Flandrin G, Schaefer H-E, Sandberg AA, Kanfer EJ. *An Atlas of Malignant Haematology*; Martin Dunitz: London 1996 for Figure 4.6

New England Journal of Medicine for Figures 3.9, 5.14, 5.21, 7.1, 7.2, 7.5, 8.2, 8.3, 9.14, 9.15, 9.16

Rozenberg G. *Microscopic Haematology: a practical guide for the laboratory (2nd edition)*; Martin Dunitz: London 2003 for Figures 2.4–6, 2.8, 2.10, 3.3, 4.1–5, 4.7–9, 4.11–3, 4.19–21, 4.23, 5.10, 5.12, 5.17, 5.18, 5.26, and 5.27

Preface

This book is intended for a varied informed audience, including patients and their families and friends, non-specialist physicians, junior specialist physicians, medical and nursing students and, indeed, all members of the heath discipline. Members of the general public who would like to learn about blood cancers should also find it helpful. We have therefore had to walk a narrow path, avoiding, on the one hand, confusing medical jargon and unwarranted assumptions about the level of familiarity of the reader and, on the other hand, oversimplification. We have endeavored not to sacrifice scientific accuracy for clarity nor vice versa.

Some patients or their families and friends may find our detailed descriptions of the disease and treatments excessive, cold and clinical, but we sincerely believe that most will benefit from understanding not only what is being done but also why it is being done. This is in keeping with the twenty-first century view that patients and their partners and families should be active participants in their medical care and probably shun the past paternalistic attitude. The internet-led explosion over the past decade has filled much of the vacuum created by specialist physicians (much of it, probably, inadvertently), but this has sadly become a daunting challenge to navigate, even for the specialist.

The Web illustrates much on the disease and treatments, even elegantly with yet more letters in the alphabet cocktail of the combination treatments, and subsequent information detailing even more aggressive attacks on the bone marrow, with or without stem cell support. A senior specialist colleague and friend recently confided that some of the Web-generated information would not encourage him to approach blood cancer, if he acquired it, with anything other than terror. We hope the readers of this book will appreciate our voices and, importantly, we hope to make their journeys easier.

TM
JG
SM

Figures

Tables

Abbreviations

ALL	Acute lymphoblastic leukemia
Allo	Allogeneic
AML	Acute myeloid leukemia
APL	Acute promyelocytic leukemia
ATLL	Adult T-cell leukemia/lymphoma
Auto	Autologous
CLL	Chronic lymphocytic leukemia
CML	Chronic myeloid leukemia
CNS	Central nervous system
DLI	Donor lymphocyte infusions
GvHD	Graft-versus-host disease
GvL	Graft versus leukemia
GvT	Graft versus tumor
HL	Hodgkin lymphoma
IPI	International Prognostic Index
MDS	Myelodysplastic syndrome
MM	Multiple myeloma
NHL	Non-Hodgkin lymphoma
SCT	Stem cell transplant
WM	Waldenström's macroglobulinemia

1 Introduction

The simplest definition of hematological cancers is that they are cancers which arise from a single blood cell. Since all blood cells are produced by a process called hemopoiesis ('haem' comes from the Greek word αἷμα for blood and 'poiesis' or ποίησις means creation or formation), cancers such as leukemias, lymphomas and myelomas are often referred to as blood cancers and in medical parlance blood cancer is referred to as hematological cancer. During our early (fetal) life, a specialized organ known as the yolk sac, and later the liver and spleen, are important sites for hemopoiesis. We discuss this further in Chapter 2.

To distinguish blood cancer from other forms of cancers, they are sometimes referred to as 'liquid tumors', in contrast to the name 'solid tumors', given to cancers which arise from all other cells. Leukemias, lymphomas and myelomas encompass a large number of subtypes with a broad range of natural histories, ranging from those which remain indolent for long periods, to those that grow rapidly and can prove fatal very quickly if untreated. In order to understand them, it is useful to know something about cancer in general. The word 'crab' (Greek καρκίνος, or 'cancer' in Latin) was introduced by Galen of Pergamon, the Greek physician to the Roman Emperor Marcus Aurelius, sometime between AD 129 and 216. Cancer appears to have been present since time immemorial, probably even before the evolution of man, as it had been noted in bones of dinosaurs and our ancestors *Pithecanthropus erectus*. It was first recognized by Hippocrates circa 460 to 370 BC. In AD 30, Aurelius Celsus, a layman, described the uncontrolled growth of cancer cells.

Cancer today is a common disease. In countries like the United Kingdom (UK) and the United States of America (US), approximately 20% of the population will die of cancer. Sadly it is anticipated that cancers will become even more common in the near future. The World Health Organization (WHO) predicts that by the year 2020, it is likely that 1 in 2 of the global population will develop cancer during their lifetime. This striking increase is mainly due to the increasing age of the population worldwide. Put very simply this means that with the anticipated global population of 8 billion in 2020 (the population exceeded 6 billion in 1999), over 20 million new cancer patients will be diagnosed each year.

Though enormous advances have been made in the treatment of a number of cancers, in particular the blood cancers, testicular cancers and several other

1

rare cancers, the treatment of the vast majority of cancers remains very unsatisfactory. For example, in lung cancer, which is probably the most common type of cancer throughout the world today, fewer than 10% of patients are cured (defined as being completely free of the cancer in the long term). A report from the US National Center for Health Statistics analyzing data on all deaths from cancer and from cancer at specific sites, as well as on deaths due to cancer according to age, race and sex, for the years 1970 to 1994, revealed a largely disappointing effect of cancer treatments on mortality. It suggested the most promising approach was to have a firm commitment to prevention, with a concomitant 'rebalancing' of the focus and funding of cancer research. This does not mean that most cancers are invariably fatal, since major progress has been made in many different types of cancers, which in some cases allows some patients to live to their normal life expectancies even though they still have cancers.

Our task in providing an optimal treatment for all cancer patients is therefore daunting. The recent advances in our knowledge of the basis of how cancer arises promise to improve our ability to categorize, diagnose and treat cancer. Globally many governments and other organizations are firmly committed to improving the outcomes for cancer patients and large financial investments are being made in cancer research, targeted prevention programs, cancer screening and other related steps; without further improvements, over 12 million of the projected 20 million patients will die from the effects of their cancers. Cancer is among the most significant recipients of healthcare spending in the US, with the National Institutes of Health estimating its costs in 2002 at $171.6 billion, of which nearly $61 billion was attributed to direct medical costs; it has been estimated that these costs will be at least doubled by 2005. The 2004 report by the American Cancer Society shows declines for overall cancer death rates and for many of the top 15 cancers, along with improved survival rates, which reflect progress in the prevention, early detection and treatment of cancer. However, there were considerable ethnic and geographical variations, suggesting that not all members of the US population benefited equally from such advances. Sadly this is probably true for most other parts of the Western world, where considerably smaller improvements have occurred, particularly in the UK.

What happens in cancer?

The past three decades have witnessed remarkable insights into what happens in cancer. Historically, at least since Roman times, it was believed that cancer could run in families; the first reported cases of familial cancers in the medical literature (in this case, breast cancer) were described by Paul Broca in Paris in 1866. In 1914 Theodor Boveri suggested that an aberration in the genes (a gene is the basic unit of inheritance) might be responsible for the origin of cancer. Cancer is now firmly recognized as a genetic disease since genetic changes occur when a normal cell is transformed into a cancer cell; these changes only occur in the cancer cells and are not present in normal cells. The word genetic is used here to imply that genes are involved and does not mean that there is any inherited predisposition. Indeed the vast majority of cancers are not inherited and therefore not familial. Familial cancers do exist but they are quite rare and arise when there is a cancer-predisposing gene in the family.

Firm evidence confirming that cancer, or indeed the risk to develop a cancer, could be inherited has been collated over the past three decades. It has become clear that cancer cells carry certain characteristics in their genetic make-up that are unique in that they enable genetic changes to be passed from one cell to another (horizontally; somatically) as opposed to the usual inherited changes that are carried from parent to child (vertically; germ-line). More recently we have learned that alterations (cancer-specific mutations) in genes, inherited or acquired, pave the way for a normal cell to become cancerous (or neoplastic or malignant, in the parlance of cancer medicine).

Recently Mel Greaves and his colleagues in London investigated whether a leukemia-specific abnormality arises in infants who develop acute leukemia (in this case, acute lymphoblastic leukemia) prenatally (prior to birth). By means of an elegant analysis of neonatal Guthrie blood spot cards (see Glossary) for children aged between 2 and 5 years, who had newly diagnosed leukemia, they were able to confirm that some childhood leukemias do indeed start before birth. Studies in identical twins show, however, that the first event, by itself, is insufficient for the clinical development of leukemia and that additional postnatal genetic events are required, lending support to the notion of the sequential nature of the acquisition of abnormal (pathological) genes over a certain time period. We discuss this further below.

Molecular basis of cancer

A cell is the smallest single living unit and there are about 10^{13} to 10^{14} in the human body. There are many different types of cells. They have a surface membrane ('skin') which is vital for the recognition and behavioral control of the cell; cytoplasm ('pulp') that harbors the 'cytoskeleton' which is made up of a network of microfilaments in microtubules and influences the cell's shape, motility, adhesion and division; and a nucleus ('pip') that can be thought of as the cell's brain or command center. Figure 1.1 is a picture (electron micrograph) of a cell. The cell surface is composed mainly of a fluid lipid ('fatty') structure in which a large number of complex proteins are floating. These proteins have external domains, which can be recognized by the immune system from outside the cell. Internally many of these molecules connect with multiple pathways (known as signaling pathways)

3

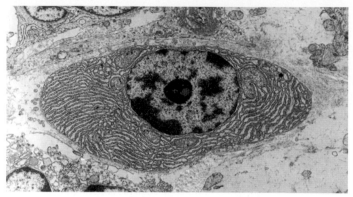

Figure 1.1   An electron micrograph of a cell (courtesy of Dr Brian Eyden).

that are part of an elaborate communications system which permits us to perceive, integrate and respond appropriately to local, environmental, and behavioral stimuli. Figure 1.2 is a simplified depiction of a cell's signaling pathways. Many of the complex proteins on the cell surface also act as 'pumps', whereby they can regulate the intrusion/extrusion of materials to the cell. The cell surfaces also harbor 'receptors', which can send messages to the nucleus. For example one critical receptor is the growth factor receptor, which can send signals for increased growth to the nucleus. Each specific

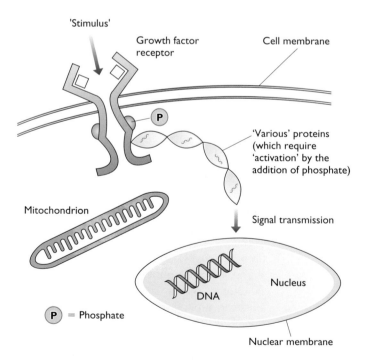

Figure 1.2   A simplified depiction of a cancer cell's signaling pathways.

molecule links only with its unique complementary receptor, like a key in a lock. Binding of appropriate proteins and related substances known as ligands to the receptors or other cell surface molecules induces conformational change (known as signal transduction in molecular biology parlance) and generation of second messengers. These messengers, in turn, activate other factors (known as transcription factors) which act on the nucleus and affect cell growth, survival and function. These are some of the basic materials and processes important for the highly co-ordinated, integrated and orderly function of the human body. We discuss the contents of the nucleus which are of paramount importance for this paradigm in the next section.

Other important methods of cellular communication include contacts between individual cells. This occurs through a variety of mechanisms and the proximity of interacting cells dictates how such communications occur. Cells that are in direct contact with each other can establish direct lines of communication through plasma membrane junctions or pores (holes) that allow exchange of small molecules or the propagation of electric signals. Identification of many of the molecules mediating cell-to-cell communications has facilitated the use of molecular approaches to defining the mechanisms by which target cells respond to signals and modify their behavior accordingly.

Genetics and genomics of cancer

Life begins as a single cell (from the fertilized egg) that divides and whose progeny divides, over and over, according to a unique set of coded instructions present in their nuclei. It is estimated that an adult human being is the product of 10^{16} cell divisions. The nucleus harbors about 40,000 tiny parts called genes. Each gene consists of a substance known as deoxyribonucleic acid (DNA), and it is the DNA which determines exactly how our bodies are assembled and gives us our individual characteristics. Much of this has been learned over the past four decades, largely from the progress in biomedical science, and more specifically in genetics and genomics, owing to an increasing understanding of the cellular and molecular mechanisms underlying the disease process. The work of James Watson, Francis Crick and Rosalind Franklin led in 1953 to the discovery that DNA in cells was comprised of two complementary strands organized as a double helix, at Cambridge University, UK. It is of interest that the first two investigators received a Nobel Prize in 1962 for this work; sadly Franklin died in 1958 without being accorded much credit for her contributions to this work. This and other related work paved the way for the current Human Genome Mapping Project, a large, multinational effort that has among its goals determining the complete human genetic sequence. The terms genetics and genomics are often incorrectly used interchangeably. Genetics is the study of inherited traits or characteristics, while genomics is the study of the structure and composition of the material encoding these genetic instructions.

The genetic information is coded by the sequence of four deoxyribonu-cleotides (adenine, thymine, cytosine and guanine) which comprise the 'genetic alphabet' within the DNA. Cellular DNA usually exists as a double-stranded helix, in which one DNA strand is 'zippered' to the second fully complementary DNA strand (see Figure 1.3). Genes have two clear-cut functions. The first is to produce a substance, messenger ribonucleic acid (mRNA) which in turn produces proteins. The gene does this when it is switched on, for example by a specific message to its DNA, and the cell which harbors it will respond by synthesizing a particular protein. The second function is to replicate themselves precisely and thereby allow DNA replication. This is a complex process requiring the presence of a number of enzymes and other

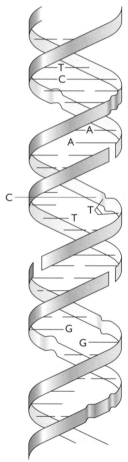

Figure 1.3   The double-stranded DNA helix. Key:
                  A = Adenine
                  C = Cytosine
                  G = Guanine
                  T = Thymine

substances. The DNA determines exactly how our bodies are assembled, gives us our individual characteristic and carries the directions that a cell uses to perform a specific function. For example, the cells which make up the liver are programed to break down the waste-products of the blood and the cells which make up the muscle of the heart are programed to contract rhythmically (intrinsic) so that the heart is able to pump blood through our body. It is remarkable that the completion of the Human Genome Mapping Project in April 2003 (by two separate groups, one based in Boston, US and the other in Cambridge, UK, almost simultaneously) has allowed scientists to determine the approximate DNA sequence of all known human genes. This knowledge has paved the way for several techniques to measure gene expression, for example DNA microarray (also referred to as gene profiling) technology. This technology has an enormous potential to revolutionize molecular biology. By analyzing patterns of gene expression, we can then relate them to clinically important factors, such as the natural history of the cancer or its response to therapy. We will discuss the current use of such techniques in Chapter 5.

The human genome spans 3×10^9 units of DNA, which would stretch to one meter in length if all the molecules within a single cell were laid end to end! Remarkably in the dividing cell, the entire genome is arranged into bundles of strings, known as chromosomes, within the nucleus. The genome is organized into approximately 40,000 genes; each gene encodes a protein and includes regulatory elements that control synthesis of the protein.

Chromosomes, which are present in all dividing cells, pass on information about the cell's functions to its offspring. During the process of normal cell division and duplication, each chromosome has to be duplicated. Each chromosome has two arms, a short arm termed 'p' (for petit) and a long arm termed 'q' (the letter after 'p' in the alphabet) (shown schematically in Figure 1.4). A normal human cell contains 23 pairs of chromosomes, including a pair of so-called sex chromosomes; in the female both sex chromosomes are designated X, while in the male one is designated X and one Y. Chromosomes vary in size with the longest being the chromosome designated number 1. Each complete set of chromosomes is called a karyotype. The normal female karyotype is described as 46,XX and the male 46,XY. Figure 1.5 is a photomicrograph representation of normal human male and female karyotypes. When a whole chromosome is lost or gained in malignant cells, a minus ($-$) or a plus ($+$) is placed in front of the chromosome number; if only a part of the chromosome is lost or gained, the $-$ or $+$ is placed after the chromosome number. Chromosomal translocations are denoted by 't', the two chromosomes involved placed in brackets, the lower numbered chromosome first. Chromosomal translocations can be primary, which occur as early as, and perhaps initiate events leading to, the development of a cancer, or secondary, which occur as the cancer progresses.

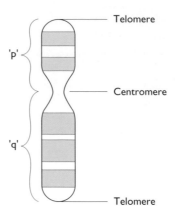

Figure 1.4   A schematic representation of a chromosome; 'p' represents the short arm and 'q' represents the long arm.

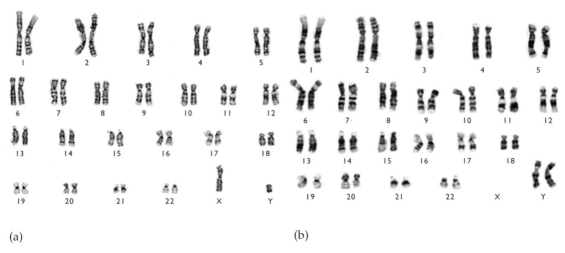

(a)   (b)

Figure 1.5   A photomicrograph representation of (a) normal human male karyotype (XY) and (b) normal human female karyotype (XX) (courtesy of Dr Marileila Varella-Garcia).

Cancer pathogenesis

Biomedical research has focused on the study of cancer with notable success. A rather simplistic view of how cancer arises (cancer pathogenesis) can be based on a consideration of normal cell fate. All cells in the body appear to have three possible fates: they may proliferate to produce more cells, differentiate to carry out specialized functions, or die at a predetermined time (by a process termed apoptosis or 'cell suicide', a Greek word ἀπόπτωσις meaning literally 'dropping off') and be eliminated. The body requires an appropriate balance of cells undergoing each of these fates for normal function and survival. Normal cells usually die after 40–60 cycles of replication. In contrast cancer arises when proliferation consistently and aberrantly exceeds apoptosis in a single (clonal) population of cells. Research studies into the mechanisms underlying the precise nature of how normal cell proliferation becomes abnormal and chaotic and how these cells lose the ability to die at the prescribed time suggest that this process proceeds through multiple stages (for example cells developing pre-malignant changes – a phenomenon first suggested by Isaac Berenblum in 1947) that involves complex interactions with the host environment. Such interactions and changes include an ability to acquire a blood supply (angiogenesis, from the Greek words αγγειο angio for blood cell and γένεσις genesis for birth, meaning to acquire a new blood supply), and production of enzymes and hormones (cytokines). These changes facilitate the invasion by the cancer cell across anatomical boundaries and spread of the cancer cell to distant organs (metastasis; Greek μετάστασις for a migration). They also allow the cancer cell to evade the body's normal immune responses.

In most cancers, a cascade of genetic alterations occurs as the tumors progress from their earliest (pre-malignant) stages to become more 'aggressive'. In some cases, the cells may be highly 'aggressive' almost at the onset, whereas in others the transition may take place gradually over many months or years. The secondary genetic changes are often associated with the acquisition of additional properties such as angiogenesis, discussed above. It is possible that at least some of the secondary genetic events may represent an adaptive response of the cancer cells in order to maintain a favorable environment for viability and growth.

The primary cause of a patients death with most cancers is the progressive growth of metastases; it is of enormous interest that the metastatic sites are not selected at random but rather determined by the affinity for certain organ sites of specific cancer cells. This concept of the seed (cancer cells) and the soil (specific organs) was proposed by Stephen Paget in 1889. We now recognize cancer cells to be genetically unstable and a malignant tumor contains multiple populations of cancer cells with different biological characteristics, including different potentials to metastasize and invade. All cells require adequate nutrients and oxygen supply to survive. When cells are deprived of either, they die. For this reason tumors must ensure a good blood supply, or angiogenesis. Recent studies reveal that tumors can influence a host of factors which in turn influence the microenvironment of the specified tissue or organ and, in 2004, we learned that tumors may even affect the genetic composition of host cells with the tumor's blood supply. These observations confirm the importance of the blood supply of the tumor.

More than a century ago, Rudolf Virchow described how the blood supply of tumors differed considerably from that of normal tissues, but it was not until

1939 that the concept was firmly established by Gordon Ide. He and his colleagues showed how a tumor (in a rabbit) would not grow if blood vessels did not grow. The notion of developing an anti-cancer treatment which worked by specifically depriving the tumor of its blood supply was introduced by Judah Folkman in 1971. By then it was becoming clear that most patients died of metastatic disease since most conventional treatments failed to correct the genetic instability of the tumor cells and the biological heterogeneity of the tumor. In 2003 several new agents targeting the tumor blood supply were introduced into the clinic. We discuss some of these agents, such as thalidomide, which have met qualified success in the treatment of diseases such as myeloma, in Chapter 8.

We have also learned that one mechanism that leads to the death of a normal cell is normal progressive erosion of the structure that caps the ends of chromosomes, called the telomere (from the Greek word τέλος telos, meaning end, and μέρος, meros, meaning a component), that occurs each time a cell divides. Cancer cells, unlike the normal cells, appear to have a repair mechanism which allows them to repair the eroded telomeres and therefore avoid death! This is probably because in most cancers an enzyme called telomerase, which by controlling the activity of the telomere is an essential component of the body's control system that prevents cells from continuing to multiply out of control, is reactivated. Normally this enzyme is switched off after birth. It should be clear that we are only just beginning to identify, let alone comprehend, the different components and interactions; for example, very little is known about the control systems that tell a normal cell when to divide and when not to divide, but the future holds great promise.

It has been these efforts which led to the discovery of the genes that normally regulate cell behavior and have the potential to contribute to cancerous (neoplastic) transformation when they go awry. Cancer cells differ from their normal counterparts by their ability to grow, divide and invade, without the normal restraining forces operating. Rather perversely, cancer cells resemble fetal (embryonic) cells which are undifferentiated (not committed) and exhibit similar properties. Cytoskeletal disruption is a common observation in cancer cells, although its precise cause remains unclear. Cancer cells also exhibit a number of abnormalities of the various cell surface molecules and the signaling pathways. The surface receptors can be abnormal or even be increased in quantity and have the potential to switch on abnormal and uncontrolled growth.

The modern concept of how cancer arises is shown schematically in Figure 1.6. Despite the stark fact that there are over a hundred different varieties of cancers, the fundamental processes that result in these cancers appear to be remarkably similar. It seems that a cell becomes cancerous when an abnormality (a cancer-specific mutation) develops in one of the 30,000 functional genes. The gene with the cancer-specific mutation, often in small discrete sequences of DNA,

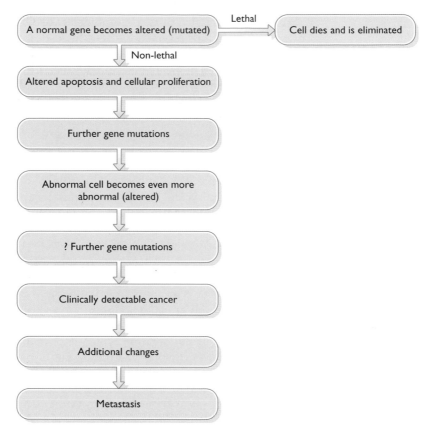

Figure 1.6   Schematic representation of the modern concept of how cancer arises.

is termed an oncogene ('onco' is the Latin word for cancer). In cellular biology parlance, the original cellular gene (which becomes an oncogene on developing mutations) is sometimes referred to as a proto-oncogene. Subsequently when this oncogene is switched on, it will result in the production of an abnormal (mutated) protein (termed oncoprotein), which alters the cell's potential to divide, usually by increasing its proliferation. Oncogenes were first discovered as the transforming (from normal to cancerous) elements (v-oncs) of acutely transforming retroviruses. These viruses cause cancers in animals but have not been associated with cancers in humans. Oncogenes tend to be named after the mammalian species in which virus-induced tumors were first reported. The evidence that oncogenes are involved in human cancer is strengthened by the determination of the oncogene products. For example, the oncogene ERB-B has been found to have homology to epidermal growth factor receptor, which plays an important role in breast cancer; another oncogene MYC is implicated in growth control and plays a role in lymphomas and a number of other cancers.

The human body also possesses another class of genes called tumor suppressor genes, which probably prevent the cancerous growth that would be encouraged by the oncogenes. These two types of genes thereby orchestrate the lifespan (cycle) of the altered (mutated) cell. Just as proto-oncogenes can become oncogenes when they mutate, cancer-specific alterations acquired by the tumor suppressor genes can also lead to cancerous growth, for example when mutations make them inactive. Table 1.1 depicts some of the cellular genes involved in human cancers.

Most of these altered cells will remain otherwise indistinguishable from their normal counterparts. Following a variable period, ranging from a few months to several years, further mutations occur within the altered oncogene. This results in a further change in the cell's growth, often resulting in an abnormal appearance. Many such abnormal cells remain 'contained' by the body's defense mechanisms, but ultimately they may acquire additional abnormalities as a consequence of further gene mutations, and it then becomes apparent to the clinician that they are cancerous.

Once the cancer cell growth continues unchecked, the cells become matted together and form a lump (referred to as a tumor). This not only disturbs the normal function of the organ in which it started, but can also invade surrounding organs. Portions of the tumor can also escape and travel via the

Table 1.1 Some of the oncogenes involved in human cancers			
Gene	**Cancer**	**Amplification**	**Rearrangement**
MYC	Breast	Yes	
	Burkitt's lymphoma		Yes
	Stomach	Yes	
N-*MYC*	Neuroblastoma	Yes	
	Retinoblastoma	Yes	
	Acute promyelocytic leukemia	Yes	
	Breast	Yes	
	Lung	Yes	
ABL	Chronic myeloid leukemia		Yes
MYB	Acute myeloid leukemia		Yes
	Colon	Yes	
ERB-B	Breast	Yes	
	Glioma	Yes	
ERB-B2	Breast	Yes	

blood or lymphatic vessels to other sites in the body, where they can grow and form new tumors (a metastasis; described above). Occasionally, a metastasis will be mistaken for the primary tumor if, for some reason, the parent tumor (true primary) has escaped detection.

Cell cycle

In order to understand how the natural cycle of the cells is perturbed by the acquisition of the various cancer-specific abnormalities in activating the stimulatory genes (oncogenes) and the inhibitory genes (tumor suppressor), we should understand the phases through which a cell passes as it divides. The cell cycle, shown schematically in Figure 1.7, consists of four well characterized stages (or phases), which are defined biochemically, morphologically, and on the basis of the cellular DNA content. During the first stage, known as the G_1 phase (the G_1 stands for gap 1), the cell increases in size and prepares to duplicate its DNA, which will occur in the second stage, known as the S phase (the S stands for synthesis). During the S phase, the cellular DNA is duplicated on a wholesale scale and a complete copy of the chromosome complement is made. The cell then enters the third stage, termed the G_2 phase (the G_2 stands for gap 2) during which the cell prepares itself for division. The cell divides when it enters the fourth and final stage, a period of nuclear and cell division, termed the M phase (the M stands for mitosis, from the Greek word μίτωσις meaning division). During the M phase, each cell divides (in half) to produce two daughter cells, each of which is endowed with a complete set of chromosomes. Each daughter cell then usually enters the first stage (G_1) and the cycle is repeated thereafter. Alternatively, the daughter cells have the option of stepping 'out of cycle' either temporarily or permanently. This latter phase is termed G_0, when cells rest completely. It is

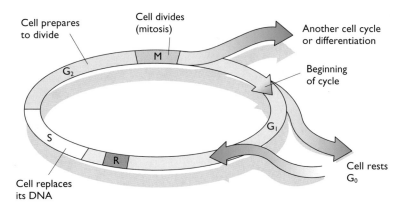

Figure 1.7   A schematic representation of the cell cycle. G_0 = 'Cells out of cell cycle'; G_1 = Gap 1; S = Synthesis. G_2 = Gap 2; M = Mitosis; R = 'Restriction' or decision point.

13

notable that the durations, of S, G_2 and M phases tend to be relatively constant, in contrast to that of G_1, which can be highly variable depending on the cell type and the host environment.

We now know that the cell cycle clock and cancerous growth are intimately linked. Independently of the various cancer-specific gene mutations, the cell cycle clock can become deregulated by an alteration of the various growth factors and other proteins and small molecules which are essential for an orderly and timely operation of the clock. There appear to be a number of crucial points, particularly when the cell cycle progresses from the G_1 phase to the S phase. It is here that a cell decides either to proceed further in the cycle or stop cycling and enter the G_0 phase. This 'decision point' is termed 'restriction point' or R, and appears to be analogous to a 'light switch'. We are now aware of a series of proteins, which appear to have an important role in the operation of this 'switch'. These proteins are divided broadly into two groups: the stimulatory proteins, such as protein 62 (p62) and the inhibitory proteins, such as protein 53 (p53) and protein 16 (p16). In general, when the cell cycle clock is disrupted, the cell proliferates excessively. Apoptosis (cell suicide), discussed above, is the body's attempt to prevent the uncontrolled proliferation. Cancer cells are able to circumvent this defense mechanism by several means.

Leukemias, lymphomas and myelomas

In Chapter 3 we will discuss what specifically happens in the origin of leukemias (referred to as *leukemogenesis*), lymphomas and myelomas. Leukemia is a cancer that starts in the bone marrow and manifests itself in the blood; lymphoma can originate in the bone marrow, thymus or the lymphatic system and myeloma arises from the antibody-producing B lymphocytes called plasma cells. This is in contrast to the most common form of cancer, a carcinoma, which typically arises from the epithelial tissues. There are several different kinds of leukemias and lymphomas. Each one is a distinct disease, affecting different age groups, having a unique natural history, requiring different forms of treatments and, indeed, having different outcomes. Myelomas result from the uncontrolled growth of plasma cell in the bone marrow. If we are to understand these blood cancers, we must have some knowledge of the normal components of the blood and the process by which they are made, which we discuss in the next chapter.

2 *Hemopoiesis and blood cells*

Introduction

Hemopoiesis is the process whereby blood cells are made. After birth, all normal hemopoiesis depends on the production of blood cells from their recognizable precursors in the bone marrow, their survival in the vasculature, and their demise in the spleen, liver, lung and the marrow itself. In infants and children, hemopoietic marrow or 'red' marrow is found throughout the skeleton (the bones of the central skeleton and, to a lesser extent, the upper arm and upper leg consist of thick, hard bone, the cortex; inside there is the spongy bone, the cavities of which are filled with 'red' marrow), in contrast to adults where it is limited to the central skeleton and parts of the long bones (Figure 2.1). It is of interest that there is an almost identical amount of hemopoietic marrow in the infant and adult despite an almost fivefold disparity in body weight! As the child gets older, much of the marrow space is filled with fat cells.

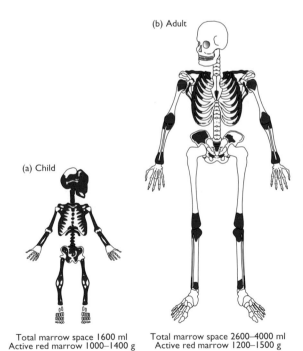

(b) Adult

(a) Child

Total marrow space 1600 ml
Active red marrow 1000–1400 g

Total marrow space 2600–4000 ml
Active red marrow 1200–1500 g

Figure 2.1   A diagrammatic representation of the sites of hemopoietic marrow or 'red' marrow in (a) infants and children and (b) adults.

Hemopoiesis, stem cells and progenitor cells

To the naked eye, bone marrow looks like jelly, but under the microscope it can be seen to be interspersed with cells that will eventually become blood cells, all in various stages of development. Although mature red blood cells, white blood cells and platelets are also present in the marrow, the most important marrow cells are stem cells, the parents and grandparents of blood cells, which maintain blood production, or hemopoiesis (Figure 2.2). The progression from hemopoietic stem cell (or just stem cells as they are typically known) to the release of the mature red blood cell, white blood cell or platelet into the bloodstream takes about 10–14 days. Stem and progenitor cells also circulate in the peripheral blood, though in very small numbers. It was this observation which paved the way for a particular form of stem cell transplant therapy, which we discuss in Chapter 9.

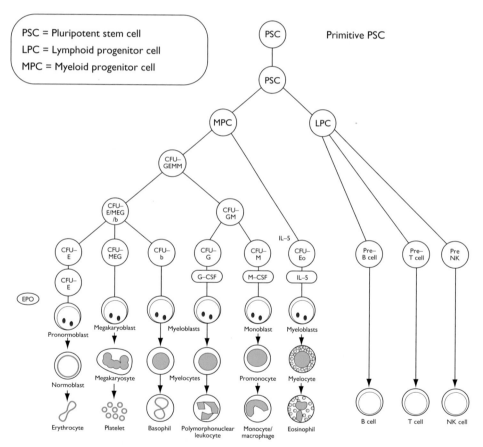

PSC = Pluripotent stem cell
LPC = Lymphoid progenitor cell
MPC = Myeloid progenitor cell

Figure 2.2   A schematic representation of hemopoiesis showing the points of action of erythropoietin (EPO), granulocyte colony stimulating factor (GCSF) and granulocyte-macrophage colony stimulating factor (GM-CSF).

The common pluripotent stem cell in the bone marrow has the capacity to replicate, proliferate and differentiate to increasingly specialized progenitor (parent) cells, which, after many cell divisions within the marrow, form mature red blood cells, white blood cells and platelets. The earliest recognizable red blood cell precursor is a pronormoblast and the earliest granulocyte and monocyte precursor is a myeloblast. An early lineage division is between progenitors for the lymphoid and myeloid cells. Stem and progenitor cells cannot be recognized morphologically; they resemble lymphocytes. Progenitor cells can be detected by special techniques in the laboratory – using assays in which they are cultured in a special medium, in a similar way to culturing bacteria. In such assays, the progenitor cells form 'colonies', or clumps of cells, which show differentiation towards a particular cell lineage, for example colony-forming units for granulocytes and monocytes (CFU-GM), or for red blood cells, 'burst-forming' erythroid units (BFU-E) and colony-forming units for erythroid cells (CFU-E). The bone marrow also contains a host of other cells, which make up the 'stroma'. Such cells include fibroblasts, endothelial cells, macrophages, fat cells and dendritic cells, which play a critical role in the body's immune response to certain alien materials (antigens). These latter cells play an important role in stem cell therapy.

Plasticity of stem cells

A very recent observation, which surprised many scientists and blood specialists, was the demonstration that the pluripotent stem cells exhibited 'plasticity' (ability to differentiate into non-hematological cells). Stem cell transplant animal models, using genetically marked bone marrow, showed that the donor cells can migrate into areas of damaged muscle, differentiate into muscle-progenitor cells (myogenic cells), and help in repair and regeneration of the damaged muscles. Similar observations have been made using a mouse brain model, which demonstrated that the hemopoietic progenitor stem cells could differentiate into brain (glial) cells, and a damaged liver mouse model suggested differentiation into liver cells (hepatocytes). It will be truly remarkable, and therapeutically most useful, if these observations can be adapted successfully for clinical use for humans.

Christopher Cogle and his colleagues from Gainesville, Florida in 2004 reported a retrospective study in which autopsy (post-mortem) specimens from three women who underwent stem cell transplantation for leukemia using hemopoietic stem cells from their brothers, up to 6 years before death. In all three stem cell recipients, the brain cells showed a Y chromosome. The findings of a male sex chromosome in the brain cells (neurons) supports the concept that bone marrow cells can migrate to the brain and transform into neural cells. Such cells could therefore participate in the repair of brain tissue!

Hemopoietic growth factors

Hemopoiesis is regulated by a variety of specialized proteins called hemopoietic growth factors, which usually act in synergy with each other. The bone marrow stromal cells, some T lymphocytes, the liver and the kidney produce these growth factors. These proteins are very potent stimuli and act diversely mainly on the receptors on the surface of the stem cells, as well as the mature cells. Some, like the stem cell factor (SCF), act exclusively on the pluripotent stem cells; others, such as interleukin-3 (IL-3), interleukin-4 (IL-4), interleukin-6 (IL-6) and granulocyte–macrophage colony-stimulating factor (GM-CSF), act mainly on the early progenitor cells. Others, such as granulocyte colony-stimulating factor (G-CSF), erythropoietin (EPO) and thrombopoietin act on committed progenitor cells. Some of these growth factors have been produced commercially by recombinant DNA technology and are now used successfully in the clinic for correction of cytopenias. For example G-CSF is useful in treating granulocytopenia (neutropenia) and EPO in treating anemia. We will discuss these aspects further in Chapter 7.

The hemopoietic growth factors, by binding with the cell surface receptors, are also able to initiate a variety of intracellular reactions. For example they are able to inhibit programmed cell death or cell suicide (apoptosis) and to stimulate cell proliferation (growth) and differentiation (specialization) by sending messages through the signaling pathways.

Components of the blood

An adult man has about 4 liters of blood in his body; women and children have somewhat less in proportion to their size. Blood consists of yellow fluid, plasma, in which are suspended three major types of cells – red blood cells, white blood cells and platelets. Red blood cells (erythrocytes) are disc-shaped with a shallow concavity on both large surfaces. Figure 2.3 shows an electron micrograph of a normal red blood cell. They contain a fluid, which is rich in enzymes and a red pigment called hemoglobin. The main function of the red blood cells is to carry inhaled oxygen from the lungs to the tissues, where it is used to release stored energy. Carbon dioxide, produced in the tissues, is carried by the red cells to the lungs, where it is exhaled from the body. There are about 4 to 5.6×10^{12}/liter red blood cells in the blood in females and about 4.5 to 6.5×10^{12}/liter in males. It is the great number of red blood cells that gives blood its characteristic red color. The production of red blood cells is under the control of the protein erythropoietin (EPO). It is produced in the kidneys (90%), liver and other organs. Red blood cells have a lifespan of up to 120 days, after which time they die of senescence.

Far less numerous but much more specialized in their function are the white blood cells (leukocytes). The blood contains about 4 to 10×10^{9}/liter leukocytes.

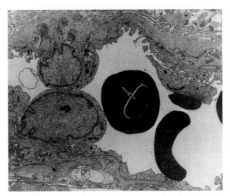

Figure 2.3   An electron micrograph of a normal red blood cell (courtesy of Dr Brian Eyden).

There are three major types of leukocytes – granulocytes, monocytes and lymphocytes; there are three types of polymorph granulocytic leukocytes – neutrophils, eosinophils and basophils (Figure 2.4). All are important components of the immune system and help in fighting infection and in destroying alien material within the body. The granulocytes, which are the most numerous leukocytes (2.5 to 7.5 $\times$ 10^9/liter), and the monocytes (0.2 $\times$ 10^9/liter) work by ingesting unwanted particles such as bacteria or fungi and then destroying them by releasing destructive enzymes contained within their granules. Their production in the bone marrow is under the control of G-CSF and other growth factors. For reasons that are not clear, people of

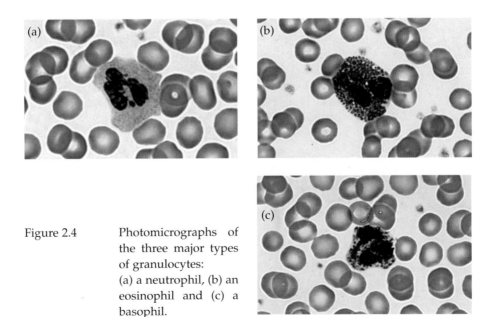

Figure 2.4   Photomicrographs of the three major types of granulocytes: (a) a neutrophil, (b) an eosinophil and (c) a basophil.

19

African descent have slightly lower numbers of neutrophils (1.5 to 7.5 $\times$ 10^9/liter) that function normally. Neutrophils have a short lifespan of about 10 hours in the circulation. Monocytes circulate for about 20 to 40 hours and then enter tissues where they mature and carry out their functions as part of a system called the reticuloendothelial system. Within the tissues, monocytes survive for many days, possibly even months.

Eosinophil production in the bone marrow is largely under the control of a growth factor known as interleukin-5 (IL-5). Eosinophils are particularly important in the response to parasitic (such as worms or helminths) and allergic stimuli. They also contain granules which contain enzymes and histamine (an important chemical for allergies). Basophils are the least numerous of all the leukocytes and play an important role in immediate hypersensitivity (allergy) reactions. They have granules, which contain histamine and heparin (an anticoagulant), both of which are released when the cells are activated. They are closely related to another cell, the mast cell, which is found in the bone marrow and tissues and has an important role in defense against allergens and parasitic pathogens.

Lymphocytes are derived from the hemopoietic stem cells in the bone marrow and also the thymus gland, spleen and lymph nodes. They are an important component of the immune system. A common lymphoid stem cell undergoes differentiation and proliferation to give rise to two different types of lymphocytes, B cell and T cells. B lymphocytes or B cells (the B stands for bursa of Fabricius – an organ which is the chicken equivalent of the human bone marrow) secrete proteins (antibodies) that can interact with and destroy bacteria and viruses in the body. T lymphocytes or T cells (processed in the thymus gland, an organ behind the sternum or breastbone), mediate the immune responses to viruses and fungi and also help the B lymphocytes (this subset is called T-helper cell). The majority of peripheral blood lymphocytes are T cells (70%) (Figure 2.5). The B cells mature primarily in the bone marrow, in contrast to the T cells, which mature in the thymus gland, and to a lesser extent, the lymph nodes, liver, spleen and the reticuloendothelial system (see monocytes, above).

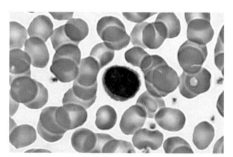

Figure 2.5   A photomicrograph of a normal lymphocyte.

The third type of cell in the blood is the platelet or thrombocyte (Figure 2.6a and b). Figure 2.7 shows an electron micrograph of a normal platelet. Platelets are formed by a process called thrombopoiesis from large multi-nucleated cells called megakaryocytes (Figure 2.8), which are derived from the hemopoietic stem cells in the bone marrow. Platelets break off from the megakaryocyte cytoplasm and enter peripheral blood, where they circulate for 6 to 8 days and are then destroyed in the spleen or the lungs. Thrombopoietin is a hormone produced mainly in the liver, which stimulates megakaryocyte and platelet production. The main functions of these tiny cells are to clump together to plug small holes in blood vessels, and to release the chemical necessary to start and maintain blood clotting. Platelets are therefore vital in the maintenance of small blood vessels, and spontaneous bleeding may occur if there are too few of them. Normally, there are about 150 to 400 $\times$ 10^9/liter platelets in the blood.

Unlike many other cells in the body, the population of blood cells is not fixed; blood cells are released from the bone marrow into the blood, where they

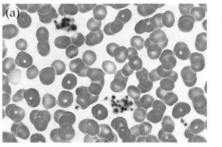 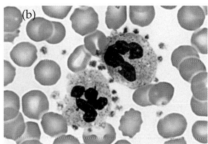

Figure 2.6   A photomicrograph of (a) normal platelet aggregates and (b) platelet satellitism (a rare phenomenon in which platelets adhere to neutrophils).

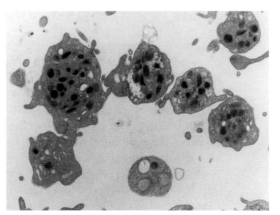

Figure 2.7   An electron micrograph of a platelet (courtesy of Dr Brian Eyden).

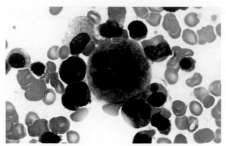

Figure 2.8   A photomicrograph of a normal megakaryocyte surrounded by smaller cells.

circulate until they die. It is therefore remarkable that despite the fact that the population or, indeed, concentration of cells in the blood varies widely, the values observed in normal individuals are remarkably consistent, particularly considering the vast differences in the lifespans of these cells. Red blood cells survive in the bloodstream for about 120 days and are continuously replaced. The lifespan of white blood cells is variable, ranging from only a few hours (some granulocytes) to months or years (some lymphocytes); some T lymphocytes appear to survive for the entire lifespan of the individual, carrying within them the programs imprinted on them by the thymus gland. Platelets survive for 7 to 10 days.

When a defect causes too few blood cells to be produced or when there is something wrong with the blood cells, problems arise. If it is mainly the red blood cells that are affected, the patient will appear pale or anemic. The tissues will not receive enough oxygen, and this will make the patient feel tired and weak. If white blood cells are affected, the body's ability to fight germs will be impaired and the patient will be susceptible to infections. If platelets are involved, there will be a tendency for bruising and bleeding, primarily from the gums or nose. Sometimes small blood vessels will leak and produce tiny skin bleeds, called petechiae, which resemble freckles (Figure 2.9).

Progress in understanding the blood has been closely linked to the development of improved techniques for examining both blood and the bone marrow. The introduction of microscopes capable of magnifying particles by 100 times or more led to the recognition of red blood cells at the end of the eighteenth century and of the white blood cells at the beginning of the nineteenth century. The number of white blood cells which would normally be found in the peripheral blood circulation was defined soon after, and in 1845 two reports appeared within a fortnight of one another (John Bennett and Rudolph Virchow, discussed in Chapter 3), each claiming to be the first to describe patients who had an excess of white blood cells in their peripheral blood for which no infectious or other cause could be found. Such patients were described as having '*weisses blut*' (German for 'white blood', later translated into Greek as λευκαιμια 'leukemia'), a term coined by Virchow. The

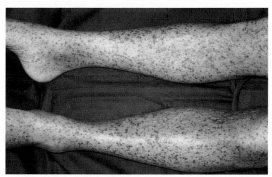

Figure 2.9   Tiny skin bleeds (purpura), usually seen in patients with low numbers of platelets (in this case in a patient with acute myeloid leukemia) (courtesy of Prof Victor Hoffbrand).

term 'white blood' was used because at that time it was thought that the high number of white blood cells in the blood actually made the blood appear white. Although this was later shown to be untrue, the term 'leukemia' continued to be used to describe this disease. Bennett preferred the term 'leukocythemia', from the Greek for white (λευκός), blood (αἷμα) and cell (κύτταρον).

When the peripheral blood of patients with increased numbers of white blood cells was examined by special staining techniques, it was found that the specific white blood cell affected varied from patient to patient. This discovery paved the way for the modern classifications of leukemia, which will be described in Chapter 4.

In 1986, a technology, defined as the 'cluster of differentiation' nomenclature system was developed whereby the cell surface proteins on the hemopoietic cell's membrane can be recognized by reactivity with specific chemical reagents (monoclonal antibodies). Their presence gives information about the lineage, function or stage of development of a particular cell population. The cluster of differentiation (CD) nomenclature groups together antibodies recognizing the same surface protein (antigen). They are particularly useful for studying the lymphocytes and have proved most useful in the modern classification of the majority of lymphomas, described in Chapter 4.

Immune response

The immune system is a complex network of cells and organs that work together to defend the body against 'foreign' material and has the remarkable ability to distinguish between the body's cells ('self') and 'foreign' cells. An antigen is considered to be anything that can trigger the immune response. Specificity of the immune response derives from amplification of antigen-selected lymphocytes, both T cells and B cells, which play a central role. The immune system's functions are largely divided into the 'fluid' component (called humoral, after the Latin word *humor* for fluid), which is made up of the B cells and their products, and the 'cellular' component, whose functions are performed by the T cells. The T-cell receptor on T cells and surface immunoglobulin on B cells are molecules that have a variable and constant portion. The variability ensures that a specific antigen is recognized by a lymphocyte with a matching variable region.

The immune response involves interaction between T cells, B cells and a cell called the antigen-presenting cell (APC). A B cell is programmed to produce one specific antibody; when it encounters its triggering antigen, it gives rise to plasma cells, which have the ability to produce millions of identical antibody molecules (Figure 2.10). An antigen matches an antibody in the same way as a key matches a lock. Antibodies belong to a family of large molecules called immunoglobulins produced by the plasma cells. In humans there are five main groups of immunoglobulins, each playing a different strategic defense role: IgG, IgM, IgA, IgD and IgE. Each is composed of light and heavy chains, and each chain is made up of variable, joining and constant regions. Each immunoglobulin plays a specific role – for example IgA is found largely in body secretions, such as tears, saliva and respiratory system secretions, and is therefore able to guard against invading antigens.

There are three main types of T cells: helper cells (CD4+) recruit B cells to produce antibodies and induce other T cells with cytotoxic activity to kill a specific target; suppressor cells (CD8+) help down-regulate the immune response and help regulate B-cell proliferation; and cytotoxic cells (also CD8+), which are mainly killer cells. T cells also secrete potent chemicals (lymphokines) which attract the various immune cells and have the ability to orchestrate the destruction of target cells. Another kind of lymphocyte, the natural killer cell (NK cell), is neither a B cell nor T cell; NK cells have a T-cell surface marker (CD8+) and are very potent killers, attacking any foe, in contrast to cytotoxic T cells that will attack only specific matching targets.

In addition to the above, the body also has a group of plasma proteins and cell surface receptors which, if activated, interact with a number of body

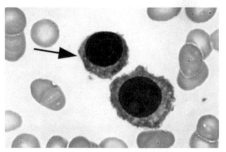

Figure 2.10   A photomicrograph of a normal plasma cell (arrowed).

chemicals and help the action of antibodies, assisting the body to eliminate 'antigen–antibody complexes'. These proteins comprise 'the complement system'.

It is remarkable how the immune system deals with the vast number of antigens every day and, so far, little is known about how the immune system distinguishes between dangerous and relatively innocuous stimuli. A very recent scientific observation suggests that the presence of crystalline uric acid is an important cellular danger signal which provokes the immune system to activate the antigen-presenting cells (see above), one major example of which is the dendritic cell. The immune system is also the body's major defense against cancer cells. When a normal cell becomes cancerous, some of the surface antigens change and are recognized as 'foreign'. This often provokes an immune response that may be able to eliminate the cancer cell. Sadly the immune system often fails or is overwhelmed in this situation and the cancer cells grow and form a tumor. Many efforts have been directed into this particular situation, resulting in a number of therapeutic strategies, such as biological response modifiers, antibodies (monoclonal) specifically made to recognize specific cancers and coupled with drugs or radioactive materials, vaccines and other agents. Clearly, learning more about the process of recognition of danger signals by the APC and T-cell priming will help develop new and better vaccines against cancers and also against a host of infectious agents, such as HIV, tuberculosis and hepatitis C. We will discuss some of these important immunological treatments in Chapter 8. We will also discuss the increasing, and perhaps critical, role of the immune response for the success of stem cell transplantation in many different forms of cancer.

The lymphatic system

The lymphatic system is essentially made up of the lymphatic vessels and the lymphoid tissue. There are two principal types of lymphoid tissue: central (bone marrow and thymus) and peripheral (blood, spleen, lymph node and mucosa-associated, such as the 'skin'-lining of the gut). The lymphocytes are the principal cells found in the lymphatic system, which is essentially composed of about 600 lymph nodes that are distributed widely in the body and are connected by an extensive network of lymphatic vessels. These lymphatic vessels contain lymph, a milky fluid, in which the lymphocytes are suspended. The smaller lymphatic vessels drain into larger lymphatic vessels, which empty into blood vessels, thereby allowing the circulating lymphocytes to return to the blood and bone marrow.

The lymph nodes are small (less than 0.5 cm in size), bean-shaped and have a rather unique anatomical structure in which the T cells concentrate in the outer paracortex, the B cells in and around the inner medulla, and the plasma cells (which arise from B cells) mainly in the medulla (shown schematically in Figure 2.11). Major lymph node clusters are found in the neck, both armpits, abdomen and both groins. Other elements of the lymphatic system are the tonsils, adenoids and spleen. The spleen is a roughly spherical organ, with a diameter of about 11–12 cm, situated at the upper left quadrant of the abdomen, and like the lymph nodes has a unique anatomical structure with specialized compartments where immune cells congregate and confront antigens. The tonsils and adenoids are clumps of lymphoid tissue.

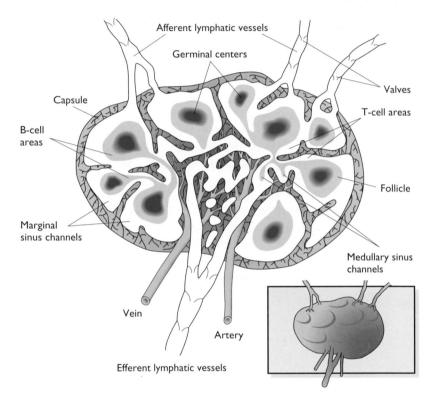

Figure 2.11   A schematic representation of a normal lymph node (courtesy of Mr Paul Chantry).

3

What happens in leukemias, lymphomas and myelomas?

Introduction

There is now considerable evidence based on molecular and biomedical studies that the leukemias, lymphomas and myelomas each originate in a single cell in the bone marrow, thymus or peripheral lymphoid tissue. The reason why a single cell is prone to become a cancerous (malignant) cell is unclear. Once the cell has become malignant, it divides and forms daughter cells with an identical make-up. This process is sometimes referred to as a clonal expansion. Why this malignant clone should escape from normal body controls is unclear, though there are a number of interesting, and perhaps competing, hypotheses and we will discuss these shortly.

The leukemias are a group of disorders characterized by the excessive accumulation of abnormal white cells in the bone marrow and peripheral blood. The lymphomas (a term derived from the Greek word λέμφος '*lymph*' meaning the colorless fluid circulating in the special lymphatic vessels of the body; '-*oma*' is Greek ωμα, a suffix that has no English equivalent) are a heterogeneous group of cancers that originate in lymphoid cells in lymph nodes or other lymphoid tissue. The best characterized of the lymphomas is Hodgkin lymphoma; the remainder constitute a rather motley collection of conditions, ranging from those with a very indolent natural history to those which are very aggressive and unless treated promptly, rapidly fatal. The phrase non-Hodgkin lymphoma has been coined to cover this latter group of diseases and, though rather unsatisfactory, no better term has yet been proposed. The name, however, has considerable historical context and we discuss this under the sub-heading of history. It is also intriguing that different leukemias and lymphomas are prone to occur at different ages. Multiple myeloma (typically referred to as simply 'myeloma') is a cancer which arises from the plasma cells in the bone marrow and is characterized by the production of a single species (monoclonal) of immunoglobulin molecule (a paraprotein; also called M-protein).

History of the blood cancers

Though vague descriptions of leukemia appeared in the medical literature in 1825, for example when Armand Velpeau described a 63-year-old Parisian lemonade salesman who was noted at post-mortem examination to have an enormous spleen and blood resembling 'thick pus', the first remarkably accurate clinical and pathological descriptions appeared in the 1840s, initially in the contemporary French literature and thereafter in the English and German literature. Various writers described the clinical and pathological aspects of leukemia and the apparently inexorable lethality of these conditions. In 1845, John Bennett, in Edinburgh, described the case of a 28-year-old slater who presented with massive enlargement of his liver, spleen and lymph nodes. Two weeks following this description, Rudolph Virchow, in Berlin, described the case of a 50-year-old lady, a cook, with a huge spleen. Later in 1870, Ernst Neumann, in Koenigsberg (Germany), was credited for recognizing the central role of the bone marrow in leukemias. Paul Ehrlich, in 1891 and Otto Naegeli, in 1900 developed various laboratory dyes or 'stains' that allowed the leukemias to be more clearly separated.

Much progress in our understanding of the biological basis and improved approaches to treatment and potential cure have occurred over the past 40 years. This progress has been most impressive perhaps in the case of childhood leukemia, which is usually acute lymphoblastic leukemia (ALL) or chronic myeloid leukemia (CML). Following the original description of CML in 1845, the next important step occurred in 1960 when Peter Nowell and David Hungerford described the so-called Philadelphia (Ph) chromosome (in the city of Philadelphia, USA) and thereby defined the diagnostic feature of CML (Figure 3.1). Janet Rowley, in 1973, helped to focus attention on the Ph chromosome as a probable clue to the molecular basis of CML. In the 1980s a Dutch research group, led by Gerard Grosveld, identified the critical area on the Ph chromosome and this led rapidly to the discovery of the critical oncogene and the associated oncoprotein, which together are the molecular hallmark of this disease (Figure 3.2). In 1996, Brian Druker demonstrated that the enzymatic function of this oncoprotein could be selectively inhibited and thereby laid the foundations for the clinical use of a drug, imatinib (Glivec; Gleevec) in this disease. Today imatinib is the treatment of choice for many patients with CML.

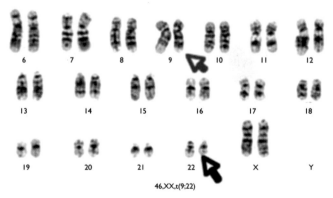

46,XX,t(9;22)

Figure 3.1   A photomicrograph of the Philadelphia chromosome (t9; 22) (arrowed).

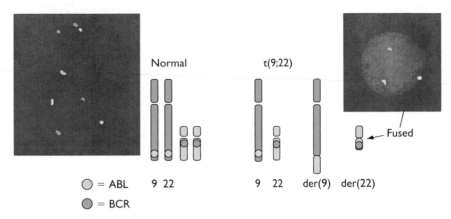

Figure 3.2   Schematic representation of the Philadelphia chromosome and the oncogenes involved (courtesy of Dr Marileila Varella-Garcia).

The first successful reports of the treatment of childhood ALL appeared in 1948, when Sidney Farber and colleagues, in Boston, USA, reported the use of aminopterin, a folic acid antagonist, in these patients. It is noteworthy that these efforts stemmed from a unique observation. Soon after the 1943 bombing and subsequent sinking of an American battleship in Bari, Italy, it was noticed that the levels of white blood cells in many of the injured sailors and soldiers fell; later it was learned that the battleship carried a chemical warfare agent, nitrogen mustard. In 1946, Louis Goodman and colleagues treated patients with leukemias and lymphomas at Yale University, New Haven, Connecticut with this agent and observed rapid (but brief) responses. There is some uncertainty as to when precisely the Yale trials commenced. They might actually have commenced in May 1942, about a year ahead of the Bari bombing with the publication of the results delayed until 1946 owing to wartime secrecy. This paved the way for the 'modern' era of chemotherapy with cytotoxic drugs to treat cancer.

The earliest attempts to treat cancer, which were largely ineffective, are recorded in ancient documents. The Ebers papyrus, the Edwin Smith papyrus and the Ramayana describe malignant diseases and their treatments in Ancient Egypt around 1500 BC. Dioscorides, in the first century AD, compiled a list of medicinal herbs and botanicals which remained in use for 15 centuries (and remain useful as 'alternative' medicine today). Ibn Sina (also known as Avicenna), in the eleventh century, used arsenical therapy systemically, although it received little attention then. Arsenic compounds, of course, have had a recent revival and are now used in the treatment of a number of blood cancers, which we discuss in Chapter 8.

In 1832, Thomas Hodgkin (who also introduced the stethoscope) reported seven patients who had died at Guy's Hospital in London from a disease involving lymph node and spleen enlargement. He described how these enlargements were primary ('primitive') affections, rather than the results of a 'secondary' process. In 1865, Samuel Wilks described a group of similar patients, and designated the condition 'Hodgkin's disease'. In 1872, Langhans described the histological features of this disease and drew attention to the presence of multinucleate giant cells, which were described in greater detail by Carl Sternberg in 1898 and Dorothy Reed in 1902 and thereafter known as 'Sternberg–Reed' cells (Figure 3.3). The current preferred term for Hodgkin's disease is Hodgkin lymphoma (HL).

The term 'non-Hodgkin's lymphoma', now known simply as non-Hodgkin lymphoma (NHL), appeared to have been coined in the 1930s to describe a related group of disorders which had different histological features (specialists now use the word *lymphoma* whilst referring to NHL). The first descriptions incorporated the now obsolete terms such as 'lymphosarcoma', 'reticulum cell sarcoma' and 'giant follicular lymphoma'. In the early 1970s, before much of the current biological understanding, it was demonstrated that some patients with these disorders could be cured by cytotoxic drugs. The first reports suggesting cure of high-grade lymphoma with such drugs were made by Vincent DeVita and colleagues in 1975, in Bethesda, Maryland, USA.

During the past two decades the enormous advances in the understanding of the immune system have paved the way towards an enhanced understanding of many of the lymphoid malignancies. The great heterogeneity of this group of diseases continues to be challenging and our increased understanding of the molecular abnormalities associated with each type has led to more tailored and more successful therapies, such as the monoclonal antibodies directed against specific targets, for example rituximab (Rituxan, Mabthera) and the application of stem cell transplants. It seems fair to say (we think) that there is no other field of cancer medicine where there has been such a bewildering number of classifications as in NHL. In the past 40 years there have been at least 10 different schemes, each subsequently subjected to its own modifications. A classification published in 1994 attempted to define lymphoma by a combination of morphology, immunological (immuno-

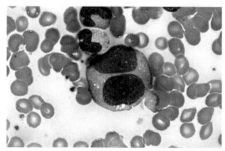

Figure 3.3   A photomicrograph of a 'Sternberg–Reed' cell.

phenotype), genetic and clinical features, and proposed 16 individual NHL, and expected to add more. This effort was further modified in 1999 and is shown in Table 3.1.

Though there have been many reports of bones with typical myeloma lesions discovered at archeological sites, William McIntyre is credited with the description of multiple myeloma, when in 1845, in London, he reported a patient with a disease called *mollities ossium*. In 1846, John Dalrymple noted that the bones of this patient contained cells subsequently shown to be plasma cells. In 1848, Henry Bence Jones investigated this patient and discovered a protein (later termed Bence-Jones protein) in the urine, which reacted with nitric acid. It is of interest that Samuel Solly published a case of 'myeloma' in 1844. The term 'multiple myeloma' was introduced in 1873 by von Rustizky in Kiev (Ukraine), to designate the presence of plasma cell lesions in bone. A few years later, in 1889, Otto Kahler published a detailed clinical description of multiple myeloma and elected to call it 'Kahler's disease'. In 1890 Ramon y Cajal provided the first accurate microscopic description of plasma cells.

The different subtypes of myeloma were not recognized until the 1930s, when electrophoresis was discovered. In 1956, Korngold and Lipari noted that Bence-Jones proteins were related to abnormal serum proteins and in their honor, Bence-Jones proteins were designated as either kappa (κ, after Korngold) or lambda (λ, after Lipari). The first 'successful' treatment was not available until 1962, when melphalan was introduced into the clinics by Daniel Bergsagel. Bart Barlogie and Raymond Alexanian were credited with introducing combination chemotherapy (vincristine, adriamycin, dexamethasone; VAD) in 1982, which until very recently was the conventional therapy for most patients under the age of 70 years. Tim McElwain in 1986 introduced the concept of high-dose chemotherapy and autologous stem cell transplantation in myeloma. In tandem with the leukemias and lymphomas, much of the molecular understanding of myeloma has been achieved over the past two decades. Some of this has already translated to better treatment strategies with the availability of thalidomide in 2000 and bortezomib (Velcade) in 2003.

Blood cancer biology and cytogenetics

The genetic lesions involved in blood cancers are similar to those of most human cancers and associated with changes in the cellular oncogenes (protooncogenes) and tumor suppressor genes (anti-oncogenes), discussed in Chapter 1. Recent research on the origin of hematological cancers has revealed the presence of specific chromosomal abnormalities in most patients. These abnormalities serve in some cases to establish the precise location of the altered (mutated) gene or genes. Current technology enables

Table 3.1
The WHO classification of lymphoid malignancies
B-cell lymphoid malignancies
Precursor B-cell neoplasm
Precursor B-lymphoblastic leukemia/lymphoma (precursor B-cell ALL)
Mature B-cell neoplasms
B-cell chronic lymphocytic leukemia/small lymphocytic lymphoma
B-cell prolymphocytic leukemia
Lymphoplasmacytic lymphoma
Splenic marginal zone B-cell lymphoma
Hairy cell leukemia
Plasma cell myeloma/plasmacytoma/monoclonal gammopathy of uncertain significance
Extranodal marginal zone B-cell lymphoma of MALT type
Mantle cell lymphoma
Follicular lymphoma
Diffuse large B-cell lymphoma
Primary effusion lymphoma
Burkitt lymphoma/leukemia
B-cell proliferations of uncertain malignant potential
Lymphoid granulomatosis
Post-transplant lymphoproliferative disorder
T-cell and NK cell lymphoid malignancies
Leukemia/disseminated
T-cell prolymphocytic leukemia
T-cell large granular lymphocytic leukemia
Aggressive NK cell leukemia
Adult T-cell leukemia/lymphoma
Cutaneous
Mycosis fungoides
Sézary syndrome
Primary cutaneous anaplastic large cell lymphoma
Other extranodal
Extranodal NK/T-cell lymphoma, nasal type
Enteropathy-type T-cell lymphoma
Hepatosplenic T-cell lymphoma
Subcutaneous panniculitis-like T-cell lymphoma
Nodal
Angio-immunoblastic T-cell lymphoma
Peripheral T-cell lymphoma
Anaplastic large cell lymphoma

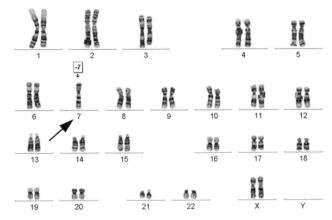

Figure 3.4   A photomicrograph of monosomy 7 (arrowed) (courtesy of Ms Elizabeth Winter).

us to study each chromosomal breakpoint efficiently and identify the disrupted genes. The information generated is helping us to improve the treatment. Chromosomal alterations can be quantitative (abnormalities of numbers) or qualitative (abnormalities of structure). Chromosomal translocations represent the main mechanism of proto-oncogene activation identified thus far. Numeric changes result from either a gain or loss of a chromosome; for example, loss of one chromosome number 7, termed monosomy 7 (Figure 3.4), often carries a high risk for the individual to develop a form of leukemia called acute myeloid leukemia (AML). Chromosomal translocations are the most common chromosomal alterations and result from a transfer, usually reciprocal, of genetic material between certain chromosomes. One of the best examples of this is the Philadelphia

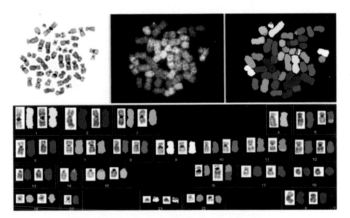

Figure 3.5   A spectral karyotyping (SKY) analysis of a patient with acute myeloid leukemia associated with t(11;19) and t(5;16) (courtesy of Dr Marileila Varella-Garcia).

33

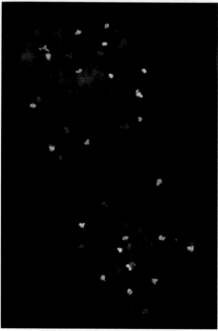

Figure 3.6   A fluorescent *in situ* hybridization (FISH) karyotyping analysis of a patient with bladder cancer and abnormalities involving chromosomes 3 (red), 7 (green), 9 (yellow) and 17 (blue) (courtesy of Dr Marileila Varella-Garcia).

chromosome (see Figure 3.1, above), the hallmark of CML, which has taught us much about blood cancer cytogenetics (the area of human biology involving chromosomes). The Philadelphia chromosome is an abnormal chromosome, which usually results from a reciprocal transfer of genetic material between chromosome numbers 9 and 22. Figure 3.5 shows a spectral karyotyping (SKY) analysis of a patient with acute myeloid leukemia with a novel association of two translocations, one involving chromosomes 11 and 19, and the other, chromosomes 5 and 16. An interesting and currently poorly understood observation is that many chromosomal abnormalities are not unique to a particular cancer, for example abnormalities involving chromosomes 3, 7, 9 and 17 are found in bladder cancer (Figure 3.6) and in leukemias.

How prevalent are leukemia, lymphoma and myeloma?

Leukemia is a relatively rare condition which is found throughout the world, although the distribution of some types varies from area to area. Acute myeloid leukemia (AML) accounts for nearly 80% of all adult acute leukemia with an annual incidence of approximately 2.3 per 100,000 adults, which increases progressively with age to approximately 10 per 100,000 adults 60 years of age or older. In contrast, AML accounts for only 10–15% of childhood leukemia with an annual incidence of less than 1 per 100,000 children. There are about 2500 new adult cases of AML in the US, about 2700 in Europe, but apparently far fewer cases in Africa; about 150 children are diagnosed with AML in the US annually. Almost 85% of all cases of acute lymphoblastic leukemia (ALL) occur in children and there appears to be a relatively consistent distribution throughout the world, although different subtypes are more common in some countries than in others. The annual incidence of ALL is probably about 2 per 100,000 children and about 0.7 per 100,000 adults; approximately 4000 cases of ALL are diagnosed in the USA annually. The peak incidence in the UK and the US is between the ages of 3 and 5 years. It is of interest to note that in some countries, such as Turkey, ALL might be less prevalent than AML in children. The disease afflicts males more than females and there appears to be a higher prevalence in Caucasians.

The incidence of CML appears to be fairly uniform throughout the world, affecting about 1 to 1.5 per 100,000 of the adult population each year. It represents approximately 15% of all adult leukemias and less than 5% of all childhood leukemias. The median age of onset is 50 years and there is a slight male excess. There are about 500 new cases of CML in the UK annually. Chronic lymphocytic leukemia (CLL) is the most common type of leukemia in the Western world, accounting for more than 30% of all leukemia, and usually affects people over the age of 40 years. It is quite rare in the Orient and Africa, although the reason for this is unknown. The incidence increases steadily with age, reaching 40 per 100,000 adults in the eighth decade. There are over 10,000 new cases diagnosed each year in the US and about 2500 in the UK, but the numbers are expected to increase as more people have blood tests for unrelated reasons. Almost all forms of leukemia are slightly less common among women than men.

Lymphomas, in particular NHL, in contrast to leukemia are considerably more common worldwide. Sadly the incidence of NHL appears to be increasing globally. For example, in the US it has increased at a rate of about 4% per annum since 1950. In some countries NHL is now the sixth most common type of cancer, after lung, breast, colon, bladder and prostate cancers. There are over 60,000 cases diagnosed annually in the US and about 7500 in the UK. Although the incidence of NHL increases with age, peaking in the sixth and seventh decades, it is also the third most common cancer under the age of 15 years. Hodgkin lymphoma is less common than NHL, accounting for about 1% of all cancers diagnosed in the Western world. The annual incidence in the US and most of Europe is about 3 per 100,000 of population each year; the incidence is slightly lower in the UK where it affects about 1200 adults. HL typically affects young adults, making it one of the most common cancers in this age group. Epidemiology studies (from the Greek words: *epi* meaning επί 'upon', *demos* meaning δήμος 'the people' and *logos* meaning λόγος 'study')

35

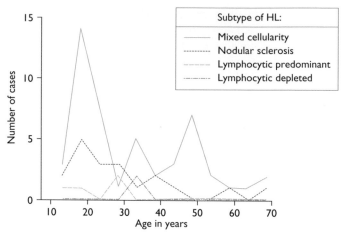

Figure 3.7   Bimodal age incidence of Hodgkin lymphoma [reproduced with permission from Mughal *et al.* (1985) Adult Hodgkin's disease in Saudi Arabia, *European J Clin Oncol* 11: 41–5].

suggest a unique pattern of occurrence for HL. In many Western countries there appears to be a bimodal age incidence with an early peak in young adults followed by a second peak in older adults, in particular men. In some countries, such as in the Middle East and parts of Asia, the first peak occurs in childhood (Figure 3.7).

Multiple myeloma (MM) accounts for about 1% of all cancers and about 10% of all blood cancers. It affects about 4 to 5 per 100,000 population each year with about 2500 cases in the UK. The incidence of myeloma appears to have increased in recent years. It typically affects more men than women and the incidence increases with age, with very few adults under the age of 40 years being affected. There appears to be a higher prevalence amongst African-Americans in the US and immigrants from West Africa and the Caribbean in the UK.

What causes leukemia, lymphoma and myeloma?

At present no obvious causes of leukemia or myeloma have been identified, although several possible causes have been suggested for certain types of lymphomas and some other types of cancer. Much has indeed been learned of the evolution of lymphomas, in particular NHL, and currently certain predisposing and causal factors such as specific infections are well established. The bimodal distribution of HL with peaks in young adulthood and older age led to speculations that the earlier peak might be related to an infectious etiology and the later one to a true cancer. However, there is no firm evidence to support this notion. Many studies of causality have been performed and some of the important ones will be discussed here. However, the most important point to be made here is that, contrary to popular myth, leukemia, lymphoma, myeloma or indeed any cancer is not a punishment for something a person might have done. Thus it is important for patients not to feel guilty about having acquired a cancer.

In Chapter 1 we discussed how cancers, including blood cancers, appear to arise as a consequence of gene mutations. It is likely that the causes of the first mutations are different from subsequent mechanisms, which lead to later mutations. The actual occurrence of the leukemia in a given patient is most likely multifactorial and probably both inherited genes and environmental factors contribute to every case. As the world becomes more and more industrialized one can anticipate that the number of possible risk factors associated with cancers will increase. It is not uncommon for patients and their relatives to wonder if their lifestyle, particularly their dietary habits and exposure to various chemicals in the environment or at work, may have resulted in their cancers. In most cases these speculations cannot be verified. The various possible pathways of cancers were shown diagrammatically in Figure 1.6 (Chapter 1).

Agents very likely to cause a cancerous growth are referred to as 'carcinogens' and seem to result in cancer by two well-described pathways. They can be 'genotoxic', damaging the genes themselves and resulting in mutations, or they can somehow potentiate the growth of the malignant cell. Based on the diverse molecular abnormalities underlying the cancerous process, it is fairly clear that the majority of gene mutations are acquired after birth and not inherited from parents. There is, of course, a small but significant proportion of cancers which are associated with inherited predisposing genetic conditions. Amongst the leukemias, perhaps up to 5% may arise from inherited abnormal genes. A small number of families with a high incidence of CML have been reported and relapse of CML originating in donor cells following related allogeneic stem cell transplant has been recorded. Nevertheless it is extremely difficult to incriminate any etiological factor in individual patients. There may be a slightly higher prevalence of lymphomas, particularly NHL, in individuals with inherited abnormal genes. Myeloma very rarely arises from inherited abnormal genes, though there are a small number of reports of myeloma arising in two or more members of the same family.

Risks from infections

The attractive idea that infections may play a part in causing hematological cancers, particularly leukemia, was conceived at the beginning of the twentieth century, when it was observed that undefined infectious organisms (later identified as 'viruses') that could pass through porcelain filters which did not allow bacteria to pass might be important. Viruses are fragments containing either DNA or ribonucleic acid (RNA), which is another large molecule which acts as a messenger within the cell. Viruses enter cells quite easily and can move from one cell to another and also from person to person. Initially, the concept that viruses could cause leukemia or other forms of cancer was widely discounted. Although scientists began to accept that viruses could, under isolated or experimental conditions, cause tumors in animals, they remained for many years skeptical of the association in man. In 1911, Peyton Rous at the Rockefeller Institute in New York had transmitted a cancerous tumor from diseased to normal chickens for the first time. It is interesting to note that Rous only received the Nobel Prize for this work 55 years later!

It is still unclear whether any particular virus is an essential contributory factor in the usual type of sporadic (i.e. primary) leukemia or myeloma in man. In the last 20 years, however, it has been established that in the development of at least two rare types of blood cancers, Burkitt's lymphoma and adult T-cell leukemia/lymphoma described below, viruses (a DNA-containing virus in one and an RNA-containing virus in the other) do indeed play central roles. In 2003, at a time when considerable enthusiasm was being generated for the potential success of 'gene therapy' in the treatment of a rare immunodeficiency disorder (called severe combined immunodeficiency or SCID), it was observed that although 9 of the 10 infants treated were apparently cured, two infants developed a leukemia. Subsequent research into this showed how a viral vector, used for the gene therapy, could have been responsible. This finding has major implications for future gene therapy protocols and supports the role of some viruses in leukemogenesis.

The risk of developing childhood leukemia appears to be increased when there is inadequate priming of the infant's naive immune system, continuing susceptibility to infections and suppression of normal bone marrow activity, for example due to a viral infection. These phenomena may provide the second and additional postnatal events, in keeping with Mel Greaves's hypothesis (chapter 1), which are often required for a precancerous cell to become an overt cancer cell.

Burkitt's lymphoma

In 1957, Denis Burkitt, a British surgeon then working in Uganda, noted that African children between the ages of 3 and 8 years were particularly prone to develop a specific type of tumor involving mainly the bones of the face and the abdominal organs (Figure 3.8). The common feature of these tumors was that the component cells all seemed to be derived from the lymphatic system. The disease was eventually designated Burkitt's lymphoma. In 1964, Tony Epstein isolated a DNA-containing virus from tissue cultured from a Ugandan patient with Burkitt's lymphoma. Following additional work by Epstein and his colleague Mollie Barr, this new virus was named the Epstein–Barr virus. Epstein–Barr virus (EBV) has subsequently been found in

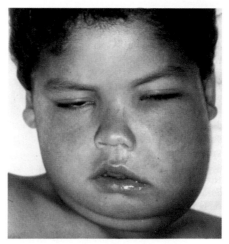

Figure 3.8   Burkitt's lymphoma arising from the jaw of a boy from Uganda
                    (courtesy of Prof Victor Hoffbrand).

almost every patient with Burkitt's lymphoma diagnosed in Africa and proteins encoded by the virus are found in the lymphoma membranes. The
immune systems of these patients also show that they have responded to the
EBV. It is very likely that EBV is one of the necessary factors contributing to
the development of this form of lymphoma in Africa.

Although EBV is widely distributed throughout the world, it usually causes
only minor infections in children, and glandular fever (infectious mononu-
cleosis) in adolescents and young adults. Why EBV should cause a relatively
benign illness in most individuals but a rare malignant tumor in African children remains unexplained. ALL has been linked more often than AML to
EBV infection and also malaria, but no firm proof has transpired. An association has also been demonstrated between the occurrence of Hodgkin lymphoma and infection by EBV. In late 2003, Henrik Hjalgrim and colleagues
from Copenhagen (Denmark) showed a definite causal association between
infectious mononucleosis-related EBV infection and the EBV-positive subgroup of HL in young adults (Figure 3.9). It is, however, important to emphasize that this finding applies exclusively to the small number of patients with
HL who are EBV-positive; in absolute terms, the risk of EBV-positive HL is
about 1 case per 1000 persons. It has, therefore, been proposed that other
factors acting in concert with infectious mononucleosis-related EBV infection
must be present to cause EBV-positive HL.

In summer 2005, Arjan Diepstra and colleagues from Groningen,
Netherlands, described extensive tissue-typing [human leucocyte antigen
(HLA); see chapter 9 and glossary] of patients with HL and showed that part
of the HLA class I and III regions are associated with increased susceptibility
to HL. They noted the HLA class I association to be specific for EBV-positive

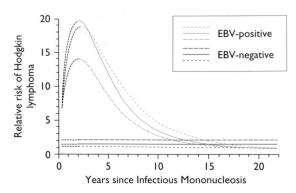

Figure 3.9   A causal association between infectious mononucleosis-related EBV infection and EBV-positive Hodgkin lymphoma [reproduced with permission from Hjalgrim *et al.* (2003) *N Engl J Med*, 349: 1324–32].

HL and speculated that antigenic presentation of EBV-derived proteins were involved in the pathogenesis of this disease. Findings from this study might also explain some of the ethnic variation in the incidence of HL. Asians, for example, are less commonly affected than caucasians, irrespective of country of residence.

Adult T-cell leukemia/lymphoma and HIV-associated lymphoma

In the late 1970s, doctors in Japan noticed an unusual form of lymphoma. Unlike most lymphatic tumors, which are made up of B lymphocytes, the unusual Japanese lymphomas are composed of T lymphocytes. By 1980, Japanese scientists had identified an RNA-containing virus that was present in cells derived from most cases of this T-cell leukemia/lymphoma (Figure 3.10). The virus was named adult T-cell leukemia/lymphoma virus (ATLV). An important attribute of ATLV was that it could induce cells to produce an

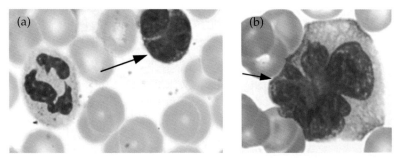

Figure 3.10   Photomicrographs of adult T-cell leukemia/lymphoma cell (arrowed) (a) low and (b) high power; note the 'flower-like' appearance of the nucleus.

enzyme capable of constructing new sequences of DNA from an RNA model or template. DNA normally directs cells to produce (or transcribe) RNA; there is usually no flow of information from RNA to DNA. For this reason, the enzyme that directs the synthesis of DNA from RNA is known as *reverse transcriptase.*

Soon after Japanese scientists reported the existence of ATLV, a similar virus was isolated from a patient with adult T-cell leukemia/lymphoma (ATLL) in the US. This virus was termed the human T-cell lymphotropic virus (HTLV) and it soon became apparent that the ATLV and HTLV were identical. The virus could infect normal T lymphocytes in the test tube, thereby substantially altering their growth characteristics.

Just as EBV causes a particular B-cell cancer in only a few infected people, HTLV causes a specific type of T-cell tumor only in susceptible people. The number of people with antibodies to the virus (evidence that they had been infected in the past) was much larger than the number of those who had developed lymphoma. Clearly, there is more to this than simple infection by these viruses.

The story of HTLV continued to be of great interest. The virus that causes the acquired immune deficiency syndrome (AIDS) was isolated almost simultaneously by Luc Montagnier in Paris and Robert Gallo in Bethesda, Maryland. Montagnier called his isolate 'lymphadenopathy-associated virus' or LAV. Gallo noted similarities between the AIDS-related virus and the RNA virus associated with T-cell lymphomas, so he called the T-cell lymphoma virus HTLV-I and the AIDS-related virus HTLV-III. It later became clear that the similarities were not as great as Gallo believed and the AIDS virus became known as the 'human immunodeficiency virus' or HIV. Current epidemiological studies of HIV-positive individuals suggest that at least 3% of HIV patients develop a NHL and the prevalence appears to be increasing, largely due to the improved survival rates through more effective anti-HIV treatments. Many of these lymphomas exhibit unique behaviors, for example a predilection to involve organs which are not part of the lymphatic system, such as the central nervous system and gastrointestinal tract. Patients infected by HIV are also at increased risk for developing Hodgkin lymphoma.

Currently several strains of HTLV have been identified and at least three of these have been causally associated with a variety of cancers arising from the lymphatic system: HTLV-I has been associated with adult T-cell leukemia/lymphoma, as described above; HTLV-II has been implicated in a few cases of prolymphocytic leukemia and chronic lymphocytic leukemia, but this finding needs further confirmation. Scientists have also reported a possible causal link between HTLV-V and a unique lymphoma, which affects the skin, called cutaneous T-cell lymphoma. Recently a causal association between the hepatitis C virus and low-grade lymphomas has been reported; this will require further confirmation. An observation linking a subtype of the human herpes virus (called HHV-8) and a rare form of lymphoma called primary effusion lymphoma has also been reported.

Gastric lymphoma and *Helicobacter pylori* infection

There is also convincing evidence, largely collated by Peter Isaacson and his colleagues in London, associating a specific form of lymphoma arising from the stomach, an organ normally devoid of lymphoid tissue, and a bacterium called *Helicobacter pylori*, which had previously been linked with stomach ulcers. This particular type of lymphoma is called gastric mucosa-associated lymphoid tissue (MALT) lymphoma (Figure 3.11). It is remarkable that eradication of the *Helicobacter pylori* infection by antibiotics can lead to the regression of the lymphoma in a significant number of patients.

Many specialists believe the role of infections, particularly those caused by viruses, may be underestimated, especially with regard to the development of ALL and NHL. It is possible that these cancers may arise as a consequence of the abnormal immune response. There are a number of interesting epidemiological studies which appear to shed some light on this concept, but direct biological evidence has yet to be established. Researchers are attempting to explain the various 'mini clusters', such as the Sellafield (UK) example, by postulating population mixing and viral infections. There are two large population-based studies currently in progress: a US-based study of some 2500 children with acute leukemia and a similar UK study, both seeking to establish the infectious hypothesis as well as population mixing phenomena and other possible risk factors.

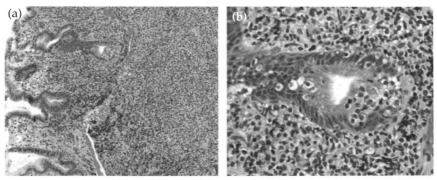

Figure 3.11   A section of the stomach showing involvement with MALT lymphoma: (a) low and (b) high magnification.

Risks from radiation

It has long been suspected that radiation may play a role in causing blood cancers, in particular leukemia. Radiologists and others who were exposed to high levels of irradiation over long periods (before the possible risks were recognized) developed leukemia and myeloma more often than would have been expected by chance. Such occupational danger of exposure to ionizing radiation is exemplified by the fact that Marie (Manya) Curie, who discovered radium in 1895, and her daughter, Irene, both died of leukemia. Studies in the 1950s by Alice Stewart at Oxford, UK, showed that babies born to women who had diagnostic X-rays in pregnancy (pelvimetry was fashionable then and involved quite high radiation exposures) had an increased risk of acquiring leukemia 5 or more years later. Sir Richard Doll from Oxford, UK, recently concluded in his study of *100 Years of Observations on Man of the Hazards of Ionizing Radiation* that the risks of acquiring leukemia from diagnostic X-rays in pregnancy is increased as the number of exposures increases.

The most compelling link between radiation exposure and leukemia and myeloma comes from a Life Span study of survivors of the atomic bomb explosions in Hiroshima and Nagasaki (Japan) in 1945. It showed that there is an increased risk of AML, CML and possibly myeloma amongst the survivors. It is of interest that investigators did not observe an increased incidence of other cancers, including lymphomas, lending support to the notion of the presence of cancer-specific mutations within the target cells (stem cells).

Recently, following the release into the atmosphere of relatively large quantities of radiation, particularly after the nuclear accident at Chernobyl (Ukraine), public interest in the issue of radiation as a cause of leukemia and possibly myeloma has been renewed. Studies after the atomic explosions in Japan suggest that a small number of new cases of leukemia attributable to the Chernobyl accident will be seen within the next few years. Some of the early deaths from high exposures to Chernobyl radiation were due to bone marrow failure.

An increased risk of leukemia has been reported in the area immediately surrounding the British nuclear fuel facility at Calder Hall in Cumbria, UK. Although a government commission of enquiry was unable to confirm a definite increase in the number of cases of leukemia in the district, the situation, nevertheless, attracted considerable public attention. Recently a French study linked a possible increase in the incidence of leukemia among young people in the La Hague area to radioactivity from a reprocessing plant. Following this report the French government set up a special committee to investigate its findings, which should become public soon.

43

Another area of considerable public concern is the possible role of low-energy electromagnetic radiation, in particular from high-tension cables and portable communication devices, such as mobile (cellular) telephones. The evidence for a possible link with leukemia is weak, but the results of some of the case–control studies do suggest a possible link with some other cancers, in particular brain tumors, and further results are eagerly awaited. No link has been established between cosmic ionizing radiation (which is greater at higher altitude, especially over the north and south poles) and leukemia or myeloma, although there has been speculation linking radioactive radon gas found in uranium mines and released from granite deposits with the development of leukemia.

Risks from chemicals

The problems of implicating exposure to toxic chemicals in the development of blood cancers are similar to those concerning radiation. Although there are chemicals that damage the bone marrow and appear to predispose to leukemia and myeloma, it is likely that other factors are also important. It is impossible to be certain that leukemia or myeloma would not have developed in a particular patient in the absence of exposure to the suspect substance. There has been some concern following the Nebraska (US) Lymphoma Study that linked herbicides, such as 'agent orange', to the slightly higher prevalence for hematological cancers.

There is little doubt that aromatic hydrocarbons in general, and benzene and related products in particular, predispose to the development of acute leukemia and myeloma. Benzene was formerly used in a number of industrial processes such as the petroleum industry, in the preparation of photographic film and in the curing of leather. As a result, many workers were exposed to benzene in the first half of the last century. A small minority developed blood abnormalities (too few white blood cells or platelets) and even fewer developed acute myeloid leukemia (AML) or myeloma. In a small epidemiological study involving 604 patients with AML and 643 patients with myeloma, diagnosed between 1984 and 1993 in California and reported in 2002, the investigators concluded that employment as a machine operator, laborer, equipment cleaner or transportation worker is a risk factor for AML and employment in a construction or resource extraction occupation is a risk factor for myeloma.

It was noted in laboratory experiments that mouse cells exposed to benzene frequently developed chromosomal abnormalities leading to AML. This provided important circumstantial evidence that this form of AML differed from the usual cases in which there was no exposure to benzene. This supported the suggestion that benzene was at least an important and contributory factor in causing leukemia. It is now believed that benzene activates an oncogene which causes AML.

Over the past two decades another serious and growing problem has been therapy-induced or 'secondary' leukemia and rarely lymphomas. Chemicals, such as are used for cytotoxic chemotherapy, and radiotherapy (radiation therapy) used to treat various cancers may, unfortunately, result in gene mutations which will ultimately result in leukemia, predominantly AML. The risk of this serious complication appears to be 3 to 10% and peaks 5 to 10 years after the start of therapy. Some of these patients initially develop a related blood cancer called myelodysplastic syndrome (MDS), which then evolves into AML. We discuss MDS in Chapter 4. The problem of secondary leukemia is particularly worrisome when high doses of cytotoxic drugs are used, especially in children being treated for acute lymphoblastic leukemia (ALL), HL or other lymphomas. It appears that radiotherapy, which is often used in these situations with chemotherapy, may increase the risk of developing secondary leukemia.

More recently another variety of secondary leukemia with a short latency, usually around 2 years, has been decribed with two families of drugs, namely epipodophyllotoxins and anthracyclines. Both of these work against cancer cells by binding to a unique enzyme (called topoisomerase II) and may thereby cause DNA breaks and increase the risk of a secondary cancer developing. It is conceivable that some individuals may have an inherited susceptibility to some of these drugs, which may increase their risk of developing secondary cancers when their first cancers are treated.

Hodgkin lymphoma may be commoner than expected in patients with epilepsy and the possible link here may be the long-term use of an anti-convulsant (anti-epileptic) drug (hydantoin) which has also been associated with *pseudolymphomas*.

Risks from genetic factors

Specialists usually refer to genetic factors as those we are born with – those dictated by genes and chromosomes. Recent laboratory research has revealed important clues which implicate genetic factors, in particular those involving gene-encoding functions relating to the genes' stability and DNA repair, in the cause of certain kinds of blood cancers. Some individuals who possess either too many or too few chromosomes, or whose chromosomes are weak and disintegrate easily, are at additional risk of acute leukemia. Children with a condition called Fanconi's anemia have inherited genes resulting in genomic instability and poor DNA repair leading to an extraordinarily high incidence of acute leukemia (both AML and ALL) (Figure 3.12). Likewise children with Down's syndrome (trisomy 21) are also susceptible to developing acute leukemias.

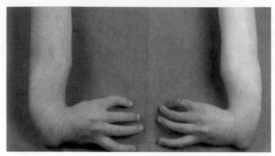

Figure 3.12   Skeletal abnormalities seen in a child with Fanconi's anemia.

Interestingly, only very rarely does the identical twin brother or sister of a person with leukemia also develop leukemia. This is particularly significant since the only individuals who have exactly the same genes are identical twins. Overall, for the vast majority of patients genetic factors do not appear to play any major role in the acquisition of their leukemia, or indeed any blood cancer. Epidemiological studies have suggested that a subtype of childhood ALL, common ALL, may arise as a consequence of a rare and immunologically abnormal response to a common infection in genetically susceptible children. Hodgkin lymphoma is almost 100 times more likely to occur in an identical twin of an affected patient, but no explanation has been found. Occasional reports of HL occurring in husband and wife raise the possibility that the association may be familial rather than genetically determined.

Risks from dietary factors

Unlike the case in certain common cancers, such as cancers of the lung, throat and bowel, there is currently no known food or dietary habit which increases the risk of acquiring blood cancer. Smoking cigarettes, however, has been weakly (but increasingly) implicated in leukemia, especially chronic myeloid leukemia, some lymphomas and myeloma. This link is dependent on the duration of exposure and, perhaps, the age of starting to smoke. Studies have also suggested a possible link between maternal alcohol consumption and infant AML. Concerns have also been raised with regard to a probable link between soy-based formulas (which contain high levels of isoflavones) and infant leukemias.

Currently there is no obvious correlation between diet and blood cancer amongst well-nourished individuals. An ongoing study, the European Prospective Investigation into Cancer and Nutrition (EPIC) where data are being collected from 400,000 Europeans, should provide more information. For the moment no dietary guidelines such as those for avoidance of colon cancer, which suggest avoidance of animal fat, increased fiber intake, reduction of red meat consumption, ample fruit and vegetable intake, avoidance of obesity and staying fit, can be proposed for prevention of blood cancers.

4 *Different types of leukemias, lymphomas and myelomas*

Leukemias

Leukemia can be described as a cancerous change in the early cells from which mature blood cells develop. The precursor cell from which all blood cells derive is called an hemopoietic stem cell. Stem cells are usually found in the bone marrow and, as discussed in Chapter 2, have the ability to develop into either lymphoid precursors, which would normally develop into lymphocytes, or myeloid precursors, which would normally become myeloid cells such as granulocytes or monocytes. It is rare for leukemia to arise simultaneously from both lymphoid and myeloid precursors. Rarely the malignant change occurs in the stem cell prior to its commitment to either the lymphoid or myeloid lineage. Once leukemia arises, it results in an excessive accumulation of abnormal hemopoietic cells, called blast cells, in the bone marrow and peripheral blood. The past three decades have witnessed an enormous increase in our understanding of the underlying process which results in the leukemia (*leukemogenesis*). We now have a much greater understanding of the molecular genetics and many of the genes implicated are fully characterized. This helps us define the overall prognosis better and allows us to tailor treatment accordingly, at least in some cases.

For convenience, leukemias are often broadly considered as 'acute' and 'chronic'. Acute leukemias are often of short duration or rapid onset, whereas chronic leukemias are of long duration or evolve gradually. Neither term refers to the severity of the disease. The leukemias are classified in accordance with salient features of the abnormal excessive hemopoietic cells (blasts). The principal purpose of this is an attempt to collate conditions, which might share similar molecular pathology and thereby reduce the effects of the groups' heterogeneity. The acute leukemias are divided into acute myeloid leukemia (AML) and acute lymphoblastic leukemia (ALL); the chronic leukemias are divided into chronic myeloid leukemia (CML) and chronic lymphocytic leukemia (CLL). The historical classification of acute leukemia is known as the French–American–British (FAB) classification, after the nationalities of the describing hematologists. This classification evolved in 1976 and was based entirely on the appearance of the abnormal cells (morphology). Various revisions and modifications made over the years have maintained the usefulness of this system and it remains widely in use. The FAB group also defined criteria for a related blood cancer, called the myelodysplastic syndrome (MDS), which has a potential to evolve into AML. Undoubtedly as our understanding of the molecular mechanisms of malignant transformation in leukemia improves, we should have better classifications. The World Health Organization (WHO) held a meeting in Lyon, France in November 2000 in order to propose a new worldwide system for classifying hematologic cancers that is based on the histopathological and genetic features. We discuss the present WHO classification below.

Acute myeloid leukemia (AML)

Acute myeloid leukemia is characterized by the malignant transformation of myeloid stem cells in the bone marrow, which are incapable of normal differentiation and maturation, resulting in 'blast' cells (derived from the Greek βλαστάνειν 'to grow'). Since normal hemopoiesis is organized hierarchically, the malignant transformation can occur at several levels and AML may arise in a stem cell capable of differentiating into cells of erythroid, granulocytic, monocytic and megakaryocytic lineages, or in a lineage-restricted stem cell. Rarely the transformation may occur in a stem cell capable of differentiating into both lymphoid and myeloid lineages and a hybrid or biphenotypic leukemia, where the leukemic cell may demonstrate both lymphoid and myeloid surface markers, could result.

The latest version of the FAB classification of AML and the WHO classification are shown in Table 4.1. The FAB divides AML into nine distinct subtypes that differ morphologically and immunologically; cytogenetic differences are also incorporated in some subtypes. The most common subtypes are M2 and M4, followed by M1, and then by M5 and M4Eo; M3, M6 and M7 are relatively rare. In the subtype M1, two kinds of blast account for over 90% of the 'non-erythroid' cells: type I blasts lack granules and type II contain granules (Figure 4.1). In the subtype M2 the blasts account for 30–90% of 'non-erythyroid' cells and there is evidence of maturation to the next (promyelocyte) stage or beyond; Auer rods are common (Figure 4.2). Subtype M3 cells are heavily granulated promyelocytes, often with bundles of Auer rods (Figure 4.3); in a variant type, called M3v, cells are hypogranular (Figure 4.4). Disseminated intravascular coagulation (DIC), a condition characterized by an inappropriate activation of the coagulation (clotting) system resulting in clotting (thrombosis) and bleeding, is common at presentation in both varieties of M3. Subtype M4 is characterized by myelomonocytic morphology and a monocytosis is common (Figure 4.5); a variant of M4, M4Eo is recognized when more than 5% (dysplastic) eosinophils are seen (Figure 4.6). Two variants of subtype M5 are recognized: M5a, in which more than 80% of the 'non-erythroid' cells are monoblasts and M5b, in which less than 80% of the 'non-erythroid' cells are monoblasts (Figure 4.7a and b). Infiltration of tissues, in particular gums, perianal area and skin with blasts is frequent in subtypes M4 and M5.

In the subtypes M6 and M7, the malignant transformation occurs at the level of the stem cells committed to the erythroid and megakaryocytic lineages,

Table 4.1
The FAB and WHO classifications of acute myeloid leukemias (AML)
(a) FAB classification of AML
M0   Minimally differentiated
M1   Myeloblastic leukemia without maturation
M2   Myeloblastic leukemia with maturation
M3   Hypergranular promyelocytic leukemia
M3v   Microgranular promyelocytic leukemia
M4   Myelomonocytic leukemia
M4   variant, increase in marrow eosinophils
M5   Monocytic leukemia
M6   Erythroleukemia
M7   Megakaryoblastic leukemia
(b) WHO classification of AML

AML with recurrent cytogenetic abnormalities:
   AML with t(8;21)(q22;q22); (*AML1/ETO*)
   Acute promyelocytic leukemia: AML with t(15;17)(q22;q12) and variants
   AML with abnormal bone marrow eosinophils inv(16)(p13q22) and t(16;16)
   (p13;q22); (*CBFβ/MYH11*)
   AML with 11q23 (*MLL*) abnormalities

AML with multilineage dysplasia: with or without prior MDS
AML with MDS, therapy related
AML not otherwise categorized: FAB M0, M1, M4, M5, M6, M7 and acute basophilic leukemia

respectively. In the subtype M6, over 30% of 'non-erythroid' cells are type I or II blasts and over 50% of all marrow cells are erythroblasts (Figure 4.8). Subtype M7 is characterized by marrow fibrosis and large polymorphic blasts (Figure 4.9).

Prognostic factors

Much has been learned about the value of the cytogenetic make-up of leukemic cells by stratifying patients into risk-based categories and selecting treatment in accordance with the risk category. In AML, patients with

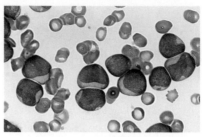

Figure 4.1   A photomicrograph of acute myeloid leukemia, subtype M1 showing blast cells with large, round nuclei and no evidence of maturation.

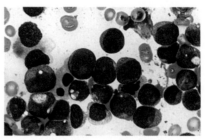

Figure 4.2   A photomicrograph of acute myeloid leukemia, subtype M2 showing blast cells with cytoplasm containing granules and signs of maturation.

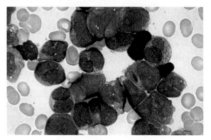

Figure 4.3   A photomicrograph of acute myeloid leukemia, subtype M3 (also known as acute promyelocytic leukemia, APL) showing abnormal promyelocytes with Auer rods.

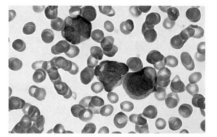

Figure 4.4   A photomicrograph of acute myeloid leukemia, subtype M3 variant (also known as APL-variant) showing promyelocytes with characteristic bi-lobed nuclei and hypogranular cytoplasm.

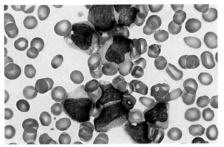

Figure 4.5   A photomicrograph of acute myeloid leukemia, subtype M4 showing both myeloid and monocytoid precursors.

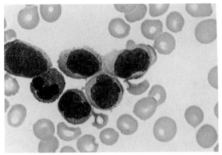

Figure 4.6   A photomicrograph of acute myeloid leukemia, subtype M4 variant (also known as M4 Eo) showing monocytoid and eosinophilic precursors.

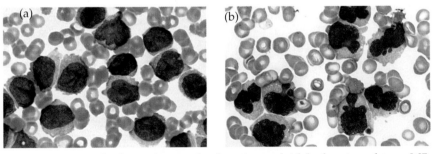

Figure 4.7   A photomicrograph of acute myeloid leukemia, subtype M5: (a) M5a showing population of undifferentiated monoblasts and (b) M5b showing increased numbers of both monocytes and promonocytes.

abnormalities such as inv(16), t(8;21), or t(15;17) have the best prognosis after treatment with an anthracycline and standard-dose cytarabine, in contrast to patients with +8, 20q− and the −5/−7 abnormalities, who have a poor prognosis. These observations have firmly established correlations between the cytogenetic and clinical phenotypes (subtypes) of AML. The implication of being able to apply this information to improve the prognosis of patients

51

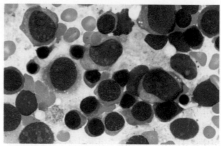

Figure 4.8   A photomicrograph of acute myeloid leukemia, subtype M6 showing increased numbers of erythroid precursors and myeloblasts.

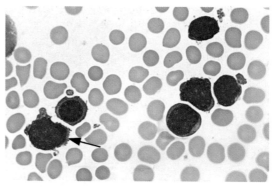

Figure 4.9   A photomicrograph of acute myeloid leukemia, subtype M7 showing megakaryoblasts with cytoplasmic budding (arrowed).

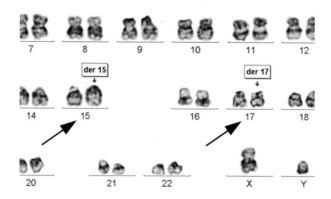

Figure 4.10   A photomicrograph of the signature chromosomal abnormalities in APL, involving chromosome 15 and chromosome 17 (arrowed) (courtesy of Ms Elizabeth Winter).

has been exemplified by the use of all-*trans*-retinoic acid (ATRA) to treat patients with AML, FAB subtype M3 (also known as acute promyelocytic leukemia, APL). In APL a balanced reciprocal translocation results in the fusion of portions of the promyelocytic leukemia gene (PML) on chromosome 15 with the gene for retinoic acid alpha (RARα) on chromosome 17 (Figure 4.10). This hybrid gene encodes the PML-RARα fusion protein and may account for the unique sensitivity of APL to differentiation by retinoids such as ATRA. Recently it has been observed that arsenic-based compounds can also exert a differentiation effect on APL cells and therefore reverse the leukemic phenotype. Arsenic trioxide has also been shown to induce apoptosis in other leukemic cells.

The good-risk category includes patients who are under the age of 60 years, have genetic evidence of t(15;17), t(8;21), or inv(16) and FAB subtypes M1 or M2. These patients have a greater than 85% rates of complete remission, 30–40% risk of relapse and 40–50% event-free survival at 5 years. The poor-risk category includes patients who are older than 60 years, have abnormalities involving chromosome 5 (−5 or 5q−), chromosome 7 (−7 or 7q−), or chromosome 3 and have a poor performance status. Patients who require more than one induction treatment to achieve complete remission, patients who have an elevated serum lactate dehydrogenase and patients with secondary AML (MDS-related or therapy-related) also belong to this category with a 30–50% rate of complete remission and less than 20% event-free survival at 5 years. The standard- (intermediate-) risk category includes patients with a normal karyotype and has a 50–85% rate of complete remission and about 30% event-free survival at 5 years.

Acute lymphoblastic leukemia (ALL)

Acute lymphoblastic leukemia (ALL) most commonly affects children, particularly those between 3 and 10 years of age. It accounts for about 85% of all childhood leukemias and is the most common type of cancer in children. It also affects adults, mainly those between 30 and 50 years of age, accounting for 20% of all adult acute leukemias. It is characterized by abnormalities of the lymphoid cell precursors leading to excessive accumulation of leukemic lymphoblasts in the marrow and other organs, in particular the spleen and liver.

ALL is divided into a number of different subtypes based upon the clinical, morphological, laboratory and in some cases, cytogenetic features. The current version of the FAB classification, which recognizes three distinct subtypes solely on morphological studies, and the present WHO classification are shown in Table 4.2. In the FAB subtype L1, the blast cell (lymphoblast) is relatively small (Figure 4.11). In the FAB subtype L2, the lymphoblast is larger (Figure 4.12); in the FAB subtype L3, the lymphoblast is mature and resembles the Burkitt's lymphoma cell (Figure 4.13). In contrast to the FAB

53

Table 4.2
The FAB and WHO classifications of acute lymphoblastic leukemias (ALL)
(a) FAB classification of ALL
L1   Small homogeneous, high nuclear: cytoplasmic ratio, small nucleoli
L2   Larger, pleomorphic, low nuclear: cytoplasmic ratio, prominent nucleoli
L3† Larger, vacuolated basophilic cytoplasm, large vesicular nucleus, large nucleoli; resemble Burkitt's lymphoma cells
(b) WHO classification of ALL
Precursor B-lymphoblastic leukemia/lymphoblastic lymphoma* (precursor B-cell acute lymphoblastic leukemia) (equivalent to B-cell ALL, FAB L1 and L2)
Precursor T-lymphoblastic leukemia/lymphoblastic lymphoma* (precursor T-cell acute lymphoblastic leukemia) (equivalent to T-cell ALL, FAB L1 and L2)
*The WHO experts felt that because of the biological similarity of ALL and lymphoblastic lymphoma, the choice of one or the other term is arbitary. When the disease process is confined to a mass lesion with no or minimal evidence of blood and less than 25% marrow involvement, the diagnosis is lymphoblastic lymphoma; with blood and greater than 25% marrow involvement, ALL is the appropriate term.
†The FAB ALL L3 category has been put into the Burkitt lymphoma/leukemia group by the WHO

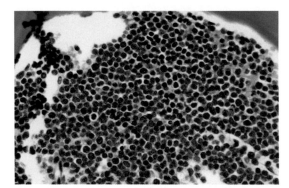

Figure 4.11   A photomicrograph of acute lymphoblastic leukemia, subtype L1 showing homogeneous infiltrate of lymphoblasts.

classification in which there is no clear relationship between the various subtypes and the immunologic markers, the WHO classification categorizes the lymphoblast by analogy with its normal counterpart in the B- or T-lymphoid lineages. Moreover, the WHO classification recognizes the overlap between ALL and lymphoma, for example the use of the term ALL or lymphoblastic lymphoma. When the disease process is confined to a mass lesion without a

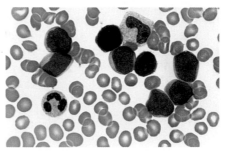

Figure 4.12   A photomicrograph of acute lymphoblastic leukemia, subtype L2 showing lymphoblasts with a high nucleus/cytoplasmic ratio.

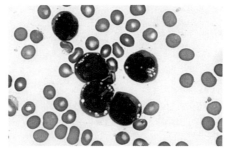

Figure 4.13   A photomicrograph of acute lymphoblastic leukemia, subtype L3 showing Burkitt cells.

significant blood or less than 25% marrow involvement, the diagnosis is lymphoma; when there is a significant blood and over 25% marrow involvement, then the diagnosis is leukemia.

The recognition of genetic abnormalities in the majority of ALL blasts (lymphoblasts) has contributed enormously to understanding the molecular pathogenesis and prognosis of ALL. Hyperdiploidy (more than 50 chromosomes) found in up to 25% of children and 6% of adults with ALL is characterized by lymphoblasts of an early pre-B immunophenotype and an excellent prognosis with the lymphoblasts demonstrating unique susceptibility to antimetabolites. The observation that about half of these patients develop additional genetic abnormalities, in particular duplications of chromosome 1q and isochromosome of 17q, has led to the hypothesis of a probable 'two-hit' genetic event resulting in a transformed phenotype which may not respond to therapy as well. Approximately 25% of adults and 4% of children have the Philadelphia (Ph) chromosome [t(9;22) (q34;q11)] and one-third of Ph-positive patients have an oncoprotein, termed p210$^{BCR-ABL}$, which is indistinguishable from that found in CML. The remaining two thirds have an oncoprotein, p190$^{BCR-ABL}$, which has a slightly smaller molecular weight. About a fifth of all children with ALL have been shown to have t(12;21) (p12; q22).

In ALL with mature B- or T-lineage immunophenotypes, chromosomal translocations often result from errors in antigen receptor gene rearrangements and so become inappropriately expressed. This is exemplified in patients with B-lineage ALL and Burkitt's leukemia/lymphoma who usually have the t(8;14) translocation (Figure 4.14) or one of its variants t(2;8) (Figure 4.15) or t(8;22). Historically, Burkitt's lymphoma was thought to represent

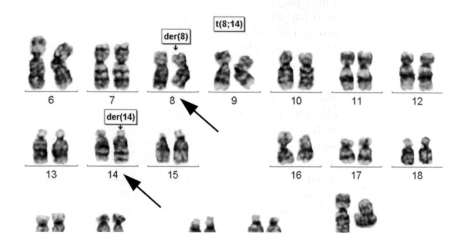

Figure 4.14   A photomicrograph of the signature chromosomal abnormality in Burkitt's lymphoma/leukemia, involving chromosome 8 and chromosome 14 (arrowed) (courtesy of Ms Elizabeth Winter).

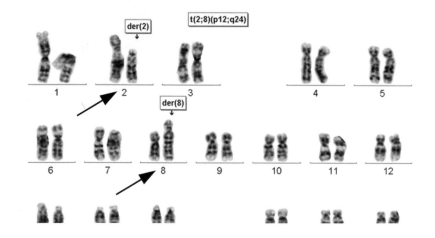

Figure 4.15   A photomicrograph of a variant chromosomal abnormality noted in Burkitt's lymphoma/leukemia, involving chromosome 2 and chromosome 8 (arrowed) (courtesy of Ms Elizabeth Winter).

two different disorders: Burkitt's lymphoma in patients who presented with a mass (solid tumor) and as ALL subtype L3 in patients with greater than 25% bone marrow involvement. However, on the basis of shared molecular and genetic features, the WHO classification recognizes the lymphoma and leukemic phases of Burkitt's lymphoma as a single entity. We discuss this further under 'lymphomas'.

Prognostic factors

Prior to the advent of molecular genetic analysis, a constellation of clinical, biological and morphological features was used for risk assessment, many of which were subsequently discredited. It is now possible to characterize subtypes of ALL into more homogeneous groups by means of the genetic features and then stratify patients into a low-, standard- (intermediate-) or high-risk group in accordance to their molecular genetic, immunologic and clinical features, as shown in Table 4.3. It is also useful to consider the degree of early responsiveness to therapy.

In general, balanced translocations in adult ALL have a worse prognosis than quantitative chromosomal abnormalities. Adults also have a disproportionately high frequency of unfavorable genetic changes and it is of interest that the prognosis for adults is considerably worse than for children with equivalent genetic changes and immunophenotype. The presence of the *BCR-ABL* gene in lymphoblasts usually confers a poor prognosis, but occasionally children who present with low initial leukocyte counts may fare reasonably well. Hypodiploids (less than 45 chromosomes) almost always carry a grave prognosis, as do infants with t(4;11). In a recent study investigating the relationship between minimal residual disease status and clinical outcome and

Table 4.3
Prognostic groups with current treatment of acute lymphoblastic leukemias
Good prognostic group
Hyperdiploidy between 51 and 65 chromosomes
t(12;21)(p21;q22)
Intermediate prognostic group
del(6q)
del(9p)
del(12p)
Hyperdiploidy less than 51
Poor prognostic group
t(9;22)
t(4;11)
t(1;19)
Hypodiploidy

comparing this with age, gender, immunophenotype and presenting white cell count, the minimal residual disease tests were found to be independent predictors of disease-free survival.

Chronic myeloid leukemia (CML)

The term chronic myeloid leukemia (CML), historically used interchangeably with the terms chronic granulocytic leukemia (CGL), chronic myelogenous leukemia and chronic myelocytic leukemia, describes a specific form of leukemia which shares certain clinical, hematological and pathological features with other chronic myeloproliferative disorders (a term introduced by William Dameshek in the 1950s in an attempt to unify the variable hematological findings in chronic myeloid leukemia, polycythemia rubra vera and myelofibrosis). The group comprises CML and other disorders like juvenile myelomonocytic and chronic myelomonocytic leukemia.

CML is probably one of the best-understood human cancers. A major landmark in the study of CML was the discovery of the Philadelphia (Ph) chromosome in 1960. Later it was established that the Ph chromosome had a fusion gene (*BCR-ABL*) and its corresponding oncoprotein was linked to the genetic events that cause CML. CML became the first human cancer in which a specific cytogenetic abnormality could be linked to its pathogenesis.

The Ph chromosome is an acquired chromosome abnormality present in all leukemic cells of the myeloid lineage, in some B cells and in a very small proportion of T cells in CML patients. It is formed as a result of a reciprocal translocation of chromosome 9 and 22, t(9;22)(q34;q11) (see Figures 3.1 and 3.2, Chapter 3). The classic Ph chromosome is easily identified in 80% of CML patients; in a further 10% of patients, variant translocations may be 'simple', involving chromosome 22 and a chromosome other than chromosome 9, or 'complex', where chromosome 9, 22 and other additional chromosomes are involved. About 8% of patients with classic clinical and hematological features of CML lack the Ph chromosome and are referred to as cases of Ph-negative CML. About half of such patients have the *BCR-ABL* fusion gene on a morphologic cells normal 22 chromosome and are referred to as Ph-negative, *BCR-ABL*-positive cases; the remainder are *BCR-ABL*-negative and some of these have mutations in other genes and are considered as having one of the variant forms of CML. It is probable that these latter patients have a more aggressive clinical course. Some patients acquire additional clonal cytogenetic abnormalities, which often herald development of the advanced form of CML.

Characteristically CML is a biphasic or triphasic disease. Most patients present in the initial 'stable' or 'chronic' phase, which in the past lasted for 4 to 7 years (Figure 4.16). The natural history involves a spontaneous but largely predictable progression to an 'advanced' phase, a term that covers the

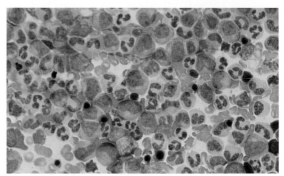

Figure 4.16   A photomicrograph of a peripheral blood film from a patient with chronic myeloid leukemia in chronic phase showing abundant myeloblasts, promyelocytes, myelocytes, band forms and neutrophils.

'accelerated' phase and also 'blast crisis' or 'blast transformation'. About half of all patients in chronic phase transform directly into blast crisis, and the remainder do so following an intervening period of accelerated phase. During this phase, there are more than 30% blasts in the blood or bone marrow and the clinical course is one of *de novo* acute leukemia (Figure 4.17).

Normal hemopoietic stem cells survive in CML patients but they must presumably be maintained in a resting state (or 'deep' G_0 phase) as a result of the proliferation of CML cells. Under certain circumstances, however, these normal cells can be induced to proliferate and this provides the rationale for autografting (autologous stem cell transplant) as treatment for CML. There is also evidence for a profoundly quiescent subpopulation of primitive progenitor cells that are Ph positive. This might be one reason why cycle-active cytotoxic drugs alone, even in high doses, may fail to eradicate the CML clone.

The Ph-positive cell is prone to acquire additional chromosomal changes, putatively as a result of increasing 'genetic instability', and this presumably

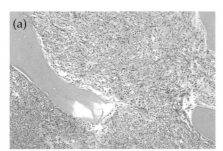
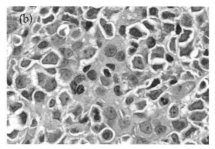

Figure 4.17   Photomicrographs of chronic myeloid leukemia in blast crisis (in this case myeloid) (a) low and (b) high magnification showing a hypercellular marrow with increased myeloblasts.

underlies progression to advanced phases of the disease. The average length of chromosomal telomeres in the Ph-positive cells is generally less than that in corresponding normal cells and the enzyme telomerase, which is required to maintain the length of telomere, is upregulated as the patient's disease enters the advanced phases. About 25% of patients with CML in myeloid transformation have point mutations or deletions in the *p53* tumor suppressor gene and about half of all patients in lymphoid transformation show homozygous deletion in the *p16* gene. There is some evidence supporting the role of the retinoblastoma (*RB*) and the *MYC* genes.

Staging systems and prognostic factors

Various efforts have been made to establish criteria definable at diagnosis that may help to predict survival for individual patients. The most frequently used method is that proposed by Joseph Sokal and his colleagues in 1984 whereby patients can be divided into various risk categories based on a mathematical formula that takes account of the patient's age, blast cell count, spleen size and platelet count at diagnosis. Stratifying patients into good-, intermediate- and poor-risk categories may assist in deciding appropriate treatment options. Clinically, however, the best prognostic indicators seem to be the response to initial treatment with interferon-α (IFN-α), with those achieving hematological control of their disease having the best survival. The recently introduced Euro (also known as Hasford) system is an updated Sokal index, which includes assessment of basophil and eosinophil numbers (Figure 4.18). Other possible prognostic factors are the presence or absence of deletions in the derivative 9q+ chromosome and the rate of shortening of telomeres in the leukemia clone.

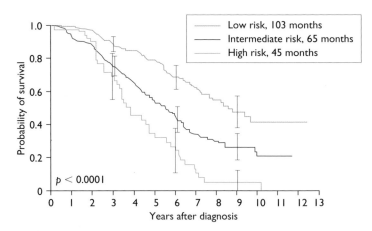

Figure 4.18   Probability of survival and median survival values for a population of CML patients classified into three prognostic categories according to the Euro score devised by Hasford *et al.* (1999).

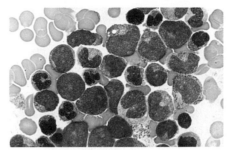

Figure 4.19   A photomicrograph of chronic myelomonocytic leukemia showing increased numbers of myeloid and monocytoid cells.

Juvenile myelomonocytic leukemia (JMML)

Patients with JMML are usually under the age of 5 years and have a disease which bears very little resemblance to Ph-positive CML. The clinical picture is characterized by a large spleen, enlarged lymph nodes, rashes and hemorrhages. The total white cell count is raised but typically lower than that seen in Ph-positive CML and monocytosis and severely low platelet counts are usually seen. Patients have a persistent high level of fetal hemoglobin and cytogenetic studies reveal a normal karyotype in about 80% of cases.

Chronic myelomonocytic leukemia (CMML)

CMML is a chronic myeloproliferative disease that was included in the FAB categorization of myelodysplastic syndromes (discussed below). It is now classified by the WHO as a myelodysplastic/myeloproliferative disease (MDS/MPD). It affects predominantly the middle-aged and there is a slight male preponderance. Patients often have splenomegaly but the degree of splenic enlargement is less than in CML. The peripheral blood shows an absolute neutrophilia and monocytosis. The absence of immature granulocytes in the blood film also distinguishes CMML from CML (Figure 4.19). The bone marrow is hypercellular with immature monocytes recognizable. The natural history of CMML is variable. In some patients the leukemia appears to remain in a stable phase for some years, while in others there is a progression to a picture resembling an acute leukemia within one year of diagnosis.

Chronic lymphocytic leukemia (CLL)

Chronic lymphocytic leukemia (CLL) or, as it used to be called, chronic lymphatic leukemia, is the most common type of leukemia in the Western world. In recent years we are probably making more diagnoses of CLL in totally asymptomatic persons because we are looking harder! With current diagnostic tools, we are able to detect in the blood and bone marrow a small population of abnormal B lymphocytes which are morphologically indistinguishable from normal lymphocytes but are biologically immature

(Figure 4.20). These CLL cells express high levels of an oncoprotein called BCL-2 (*an anti-apoptotic protein, which prevents cells from dying when they are programmed to die*) and are positive for the CD5 cell surface marker. Since CLL is a disease of the B lymphocytes (which make antibodies), it is not surprising to see a range of immunological problems in patients with CLL. These may result in frequent bacterial infections and other autoimmune disorders whereby individuals make antibodies which attack their own organs. Small lymphocytic lymphoma is the tissue manifestation of CLL. Patients who present predominantly with blood and bone marrow involvement will have CLL and those with enlarged lymph nodes will have small lymphocytic lymphoma (CD5-positive lymphomas).

CLL is usually a relatively mild disease and some patients survive for many years with minimal or no treatment. In other cases, however, the disease is more aggressive and may require more intensive treatment. Owing to these variable presentations, it is important to group patients according to their risk factors and then to individualize therapy. This is often done using clinical staging systems, introduced almost three decades ago by Kanti Rai (in the US) and Jacques-Louis Binet (in France), which we discuss below.

Efforts over the past decade have noted that cases can be divided into two broad groups on the basis of the presence or absence of mutation in the specific immunoglobulin genes (heavy-chain variable-region, known as IgV_H) of the CLL cells. The disparity in lifespan between the groups is striking, with median survivals of more than 24 years and 6 to 8 years, respectively. In 2003, a molecule called ZAP-70 (zeta-chain-associated protein 70) was found to be expressed almost exclusively in cells from patients with the aggressive form of CLL (without the IgV_H mutation), while those with the indolent form did not express ZAP-70 (and express mutated IgV_H). ZAP-70 is now being used increasingly to allow us to make better individual treatment decisions.

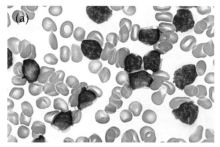
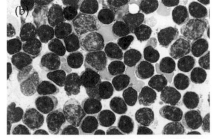

Figure 4.20   A photomicrograph of chronic lymphocytic leukemia (a) peripheral blood film showing many lymphocytes including 'smudge cells' and (b) bone marrow showing increased number of lymphocytes.

Very rarely, CLL arises in a T lymphocyte, rather than a B lymphocyte; the disease is then termed T-CLL. Epidemiology studies from the Far East suggest that T-cell CLL, which represents less than 3% of the disease in all European and American CLL patients, is the dominant form of this disease in Asia. Patients often present with low white cell counts (in contrast to the high counts typical of B-CLL); prominent splenomegaly and the lack of lymphadenopathy are noteworthy. The general prognosis is similar to 'poor-risk' CLL. There are a few other kinds of chronic leukemia related to CLL, all rare: prolymphocytic leukemia, large granular lymphocytic leukemia (LGL), hairy cell leukemia and the adult T-cell leukemia/lymphoma (ATLL).

In about 10% of patients with CLL, there is abrupt transformation to the development of a high-grade lymphoma in one of the lymph nodes. It was first described by an Austrian physician, Richter and it carries his name.

Staging systems and prognostic factors

Rai's staging system, first introduced in 1975, is based on William Dameshek's proposed model of orderly disease progression in CLL and consists of five stages which were found to correlate with prognosis. Binet (also known as the International Staging System for CLL) thereafter developed a similar system consisting of three stages and it largely superseded Rai's system (at least in Europe). Both systems are shown in Table 4.4. These traditional staging systems are based almost entirely on clinically determinable features (looking for anemia and thrombocytopenia, and feeling for the presence of lymph node, liver and spleen enlargement) and have been found to be quite useful foundations on which to base therapeutic decisions at the time of diagnosis. However, neither staging system predicts accurately the clinical course of the disease in individual patients; neither system accommodates the increase in our understanding of the molecular biology of CLL. In 1981 an International Workshop on CLL recommended the two staging systems to be amalgamated.

The Rai system has been revised more recently to include three stages: low risk (Rai 0), intermediate risk (Rai 1–2) and high risk (Rai 3–4). The poor prognosis associated with the unmutated variable region of the immunoglobulin genes, ZAP 70 and an overexpression of CD38 are relatively new entrants to the list of other previously well-established prognostic factors such as doubling of the lymphocyte counts in less than 12 months, a diffuse pattern of involvement on the trephine biopsy and an abnormal karyotype.

Small studies have demonstrated several molecular abnormalities but these have not been confirmed. It is possible that the monotonous morphology of the CLL cells may represent the result of varying molecular events. Cytogenetic abnormalities occur in about 50% of all patients with CLL with trisomy 12 and 13q14 deletions being the most frequent. The finding of these abnormalities is considered to be a poor prognostic feature. A minimal region

Table 4.4
Clinical staging sytems for chronic lymphocytic leukemia

(a) Rai staging system

Stage	Features	Level of risk	Median survival
0	Lymphocytosis	Low	>10 years
1	Lymphocytosis and lymphadenopathy	Intermediate	7
2	Lymphocytosis, lymphadenopathy and spleen and/or liver enlargement		
3	Lymphocytosis and anemia (Hb <11 g/dL)	High	1.5 years
4	Lymphocytosis and thrombocytopenia (platelets < 100 × 10^9/L)		

(b) Binet staging system

Stage	Lymphoid involvement	Hb (g/dL)	Platelets (× 10^9/L)	Survival (years)
A	0, 1, or 2 areas	>10	>100	12
B	3 or more areas	>10	>100	5
C	3 or more areas	<10 and/or	<100	2

of deletion (MDR) spanning <300 kb of DNA and common to all CLL cell lines with 13q14 deletions has been identified, suggesting that specific abnormalities at 13q14 may represent a common event in the pathogenesis of CLL.

Prolymphocytic leukemia (PLL)

PLL was first described by David Galton at the Hammersmith Hospital, London in 1974. It can be *de novo* or arise as a consequence of CLL transformation. PLL cells are larger and more immature than CLL cells (Figure 4.21). The patients often have greater spleen and liver enlargement and, interestingly, lymph node enlargement is either minimal or absent. Most patients have a clinical course similar to 'poor-risk' CLL; a minority have an indolent course.

Large granular lymphocytic leukemia (LGL leukemia)

Large granular lymphoma are a heterogeneous group of large lymphocytes which express specific immunological markers, known as 'natural killer' or NK markers (now known as CD8 and CD56) (Figure 4.22). LGL leukemia has a varied natural history, ranging from an indolent condition to that of acute leukemia. Most patients present with recurrent infections, anemia and large

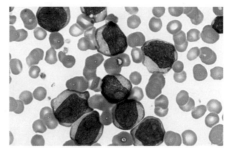

Figure 4.21   A photomicrograph of prolymphocytic leukemia showing abundant prolymphocytes.

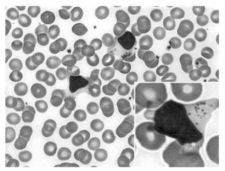

Figure 4.22   A photomicrograph of large granular lymphocytic (LGL) leukemia, insert shows a higher magnification.

spleens and usually no significant lymphadenopathy. The majority of patients with LGL leukemia do not require any specific treatment at presentation.

Hairy cell leukemia (HCL)

Hairy cell leukemia was first described by Bouroncle, Wiseman and Doan in 1958. It is an exceedingly rare disease accounting for less than 1% of all leukemias, but has fascinated many researchers and clinicians by virtue of its several unique features. Most patients tend to be aged between 50 and 70 years and males are more often affected than females. The typical hairy leukemia cell is an irregular cell with a serrated or 'tentacled' border, with a sky blue cytoplasm devoid of any granules (Figure 4.23). When these cells are examined under an electron microscope, long cytoplasmic villi resembling tentacles or hairs are seen (hence the name – hairy cell!) (Figure 4.24). Most patients present with weakness, fatigue and a tendency to develop infections. Clinically most have an enlarged spleen, which is often huge, and typically there is no lymph node enlargement.

Adult T-cell leukemia/lymphoma (ATL)

Adult T-cell leukemia/lymphoma (ATLL) is a rare distinct form of chronic leukemia, first described on the island of Kyushu in south Japan and

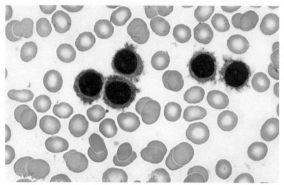

Figure 4.23   A photomicrograph of hairy cell leukemia showing 'hairy' lymphocytes with characteristic fine hair-like cytoplasmic projections.

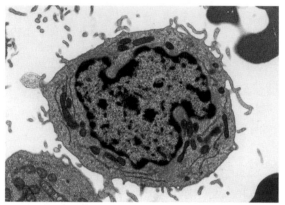

Figure 4.24   An electron micrograph of a hairy cell leukemia cell, showing the long cytoplasmic villi resembling 'hair' (courtesy of Prof Daniel Catovsky).

subsequently found to occur in the Caribbean, US and other countries. Epidemiological studies have described the causal association between ATL and HTLV-I. It has a median age of occurrence of 40 years and men appear to be at higher risk than women. Most patients present with lymph node enlargement and high lymphocyte counts. About two-thirds of patients have a peculiar skin involvement which can sometimes be confused with skin lymphoma (Figure 4.25). Another important feature of ATLL is the presence of characteristic abnormal circulating T lymphocytes. Patients with ATLL can sometimes present with lytic bone lesions and high blood calcium levels, which can result in weakness, lethargy and even mental confusion.

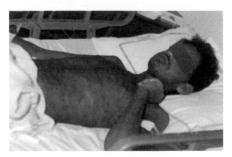

Figure 4.25   Skin involvement in a patient with acute T-cell leukemia/lymphoma (ATLL).

ATLL appears either to behave in an indolent manner for long periods without specific therapy or present with progressive lymph node enlargement, bone lesions and high blood calcium levels; such patients generally become quite ill and have a grim prognosis.

Myelodysplastic syndromes

The myelodysplastic syndromes (MDS), first described by Matthew Block in 1952, are (clonal) disorders characterized clinically and morphologically by ineffective hemopoiesis leading to bone marrow failure and a high probability of malignant transformation to AML. They should be considered as a pre-leukemic condition. MDS generally affects patients over the age of 60 years, although an increasing number of younger adults is being reported, mostly with therapy-associated MDS (t-MDS) (see Chapter 3). With the exception of the MDS with a unique cytogenetic abnormality, 5q−, men appear to be affected more often than women. Childhood MDS is rare and found in constitutional conditions such as Down's syndrome.

The cytogenetic events that lead to MDS are heterogeneous but certain abnormalities, such as loss or gain of all or parts of chromosomes 5, 7, 8 and 20, tend to prevail. The precise molecular changes involved, in particular those that result in transformation into AML, have not been fully elucidated but a number of potential candidate genes have been identified (such as the *RAS*, the *p53* and the *MLL* genes). It is likely that sequential mutations leading to genetic abnormalities are required. The natural history and biology of MDS, like that of AML, depend upon the nature of the underlying events; those patients who have a balanced chromosomal translocation are more likely to present with frank transformation into AML than those with unbalanced translocation, who are likely to present in the 'earlier' stages of MDS such that transformation occurs following further genetic events. For example patients with the 5q− cytogenetic abnormality tend to have a rather benign clinical course and only about 25% will transform into AML following additional genetic events.

The FAB classification of MDS proposed in 1982 was intended for diagnostic and prognostic purposes. The classification had several important limitations. First, the term 'refractory anemia' was imprecise and could not be identified morphologically. Second, CMML is perhaps more closely related to the myelo-proliferative disorders than to the other subtypes of MDS. Third, the use of an arbitrary criterion, for example the percentage of marrow blasts, to distinguish between an advanced MDS and a frank AML, was often misleading. This classification also had other severe limitations, in particular since there is little concordance for the clinical, molecular and biological features of the proposed sub-categories. The present WHO classification has attempted to rectify this. Table 4.5 shows the FAB and WHO classifications of MDS.

Table 4.5
The FAB and WHO classifications of myelodysplastic syndromes (MDS)
(a) FAB classification of MDS
Refractory anemia (RA)
Refractory anemia with ringed sideroblasts (RARS)
Refractory anemia with excess blasts (RAEB)
Refractory anemia with excess blasts in transformation (RAEB-T)
Chronic myelomonocytic leukemia (CMML)
(b) WHO classification of MDS
Refractory anemia without ringed sideroblasts (equivalent to FAB: RA)
Refractory anemia with ringed sideroblasts (equivalent to FAB: RARS)
Refractory cytopenia with multilineage dysplasia (RCMD) (new)
Refractory cytopenia with multilineage dysplasia and ringed sideroblasts (RCMD-RS) (new)
Refractory anemia with excess blasts I (equivalent to FAB: RAEB)
Refractory anemia with excess blasts 2 (equivalent to FAB: RAEB)
MDS associated with isolated del(5q) (new)
MDS-U unclassifiable (new)
The major changes from the FAB classification of MDS are:
The RAEB-T of the FAB is now considered to be acute leukemia, not an MDS type
CMML of the FAB is now in a new category MPD/MDS devised by the WHO
New groups have been created by the WHO to allow for a better stratification of these patients: RCMD, MDS with isolated del(5q) and MDS-U.

Staging systems and prognostic factors

A prognostic scoring has been proposed by the International Myelodysplastic Syndrome Risk Analysis Workshop (Table 4.6). It attempts to assign a score in accordance to the clinical and biological features. Patients are assigned a score based upon the cytogenetic abnormalities, the percentage of blasts in the marrow and the number of lineages affected in the cytopenia and then stratified into four prognostic groups: low score (median survival 5.7 years), intermediate score subgroup 1 (median survival 3.5 years), intermediate score subgroup 2 (median survival 1.2 years) and high score (median survival 0.4 year). This system appears to have gained international approval and should prove useful.

Among patients with MDS, those with certain associated or underlying genetic events appear to have a unique natural history such that it is sometimes convenient to consider them as separate clinical entities. These include *the 5q− syndrome*, which is characterized by a relatively indolent clinical course. Anemia is often the major manifestation but mild neutropenia can also occur; thrombocytosis is also often present. Red cell support is often the sole treatment required. *Hypoplastic myelodysplasia* tends to be unique not so much from its clinical manifestations or its natural history, but rather from a diagnostic perspective since these patients can often be diagnosed as having aplastic anemia. The demonstration of the characteristic MDS cytogenetic abnormalities allows the correct diagnosis to be made. *Therapy-related myelodysplasias* are caused by chemotherapy or radiotherapy that results in cytogenetic events which dictate its clinical course; they tend in general to have a worse prognosis than the other subtypes of MDS.

Most patients with MDS are diagnosed as a consequence of pancytopenia on a routine examination, which is the result of ineffective hemopoiesis rather

Table 4.6 The International Prognostic Scoring System (IPSS) for myelodysplastic syndrome		
Indicator	**Value**	**Score**
Blasts	≤5%	0
	>5%, ≤10%	0.5
	>10%, ≤20%	1.5
	>20%, ≤30%	2.0
Cytogenetics	Good	0
	Intermediate	0.5
	Poor	1.0
Blood cytopenias	0/1	0
	2/3	0.5

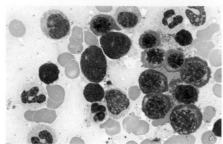

Figure 4.26   A bone marrow specimen from a patient with myelodysplastic syndrome (MDS) showing dysplastic erythroid precursors.

than a lack of hemopoietic activity. The diagnosis of MDS is often suspected on morphological grounds in a patient with cytopenia. The bone marrow cellularity is either normal or increased. Characteristic morphological changes include mature hypogranular and hypolobulated (pseudo-Pelger-Huët) granulocytes, micromegakaryocytes and a variety of red-cell precursor abnormalities, ranging from ringed sideroblasts to megaloblastic changes (Figure 4.26). Dysplastic abnormalities in all cell lineages are prominent. Cytogenetic analysis using the fluorescence *in situ* hybridization technology and polymerase chain reaction (PCR) studies on bone marrow samples are useful tools in confirming the diagnosis and facilitating classification. Cytokinetic studies of bone marrow cells suggest a substantially higher rate of cell division and apoptosis is prominently increased. Other potentially useful studies include magnetic resonance imaging of bone marrow.

Lymphomas

Hodgkin lymphoma (HL)

The incidence of HL, also known as Hodgkin's disease, appears to be stable, in contrast to NHL. A strong association has been found between the occurrence of HL and infection with EBV. Patients infected with HIV are at increased risk for both HL and NHL. It is of interest that there is considerable geographical and age group variation of the different subtypes of HD. For example, young adults in the US are likely to have the nodular sclerosis variant, while their counterparts from the developing world often develop the mixed cellularity or the lymphocyte-depleted variety. Elderly patients and those infected with HIV are also more likely to develop the latter two variants. The present WHO classification of HL is shown in Table 4.7.

Nodular sclerosis classical Hodgkin lymphoma (NSHL)

NSHL is diagnosed in about 70% of the patients in the US and the UK. It is characterized by the replacement of part of the lymph node by bands of

Table 4.7
The WHO classification of Hodgkin lymphoma
Nodular lymphocyte predominant Hodgkin lymphoma (NLPHL)
Classical Hodgkin lymphoma
Nodular sclerosis classical Hodgkin lymphoma (NSHL)
Mixed cellularity classical Hodgkin lymphoma (MCHL)
Lymphocyte-rich classical Hodgkin lymphoma (LRCHL)
Lymphocyte-depleted classical Hodgkin lymphoma (LDHL)

fibrosis and the presence of the 'lacunar' variant of Sternberg–Reed cells which show contraction of their cytoplasm (Figure 4.27). Two grades of nodular sclerosis are recognized, with grade 2 being associated with a more aggressive disease. It is more common in females and appears to be often found in the neck and mediastinal regions.

Lymphocyte-rich classic Hodgkin lymphoma (LRCHL)

This is a rare subtype accounting for less than 5% of all cases; it is also known as lymphocyte predominant HL. It is characterized by large numbers of small lymphocytes and histiocytes with occasional Sternberg–Reed cells, which resemble 'popcorn' cells rather than the typical Sternberg–Reed cells (also known as L and H cells; for lymphocytic and histiocytic) and a growth pattern which can be nodular or diffuse. Recently it has been acknowledged that patients with the nodular lymphocyte predominant variety have a different illness that resembles a B-cell NHL and, perhaps, should be treated accordingly; indeed, it sometimes transforms to diffuse large B-cell lymphoma. Clinically this variety occurs in all ages, males more often than females and often involves the peripheral lymph nodes.

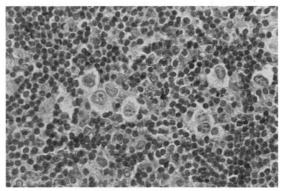

Figure 4.27   A photomicrograph of 'lacunar' variant of Sternberg–Reed cells seen in patients with Hodgkin lymphoma, nodular sclerosis subtype.

71

Mixed cellularity classic Hodgkin lymphoma (MCHL)

Mixed cellularity variety is the most common variety of HL in the developing world; it accounts for about 25% of all cases seen in the US and the UK. It is more common in males, more likely to be associated with EBV seropositivity and is the usual variety noted in patients who are HIV positive. It is the most common variety seen in patients with involvement of the infra-diaphragmatic area, including the spleen. It can exhibit a variable appearance with abundant typical Sternberg–Reed cells and an abundant, variable, mixed cellular infiltrate (Figure 4.28). It can sometimes be confused with the diagnosis of peripheral T-cell lymphoma and a rare entity called T-cell rich B-cell large cell lymphoma. Typical Sternberg–Reed cells stain positive for CD15 and CD30 surface antigens and can help resolve diagnostic difficulties.

Lymphocyte-depleted classical Hodgkin lymphoma (LDHL)

The lymphocyte-depleted variety of HL is the rarest variety with less than 5% of all cases and is almost exclusively found in developing countries, elderly male patients and patients with HIV infections. It frequently affects extra-nodal sites or intra-abdominal lymph nodes. There are often large numbers of Sternberg–Reed cells and it is a particularly aggressive form of HL.

Lymphocyte-rich classic Hodgkin's lymphoma (NLPHL)

This variety of HL has recently been recognized by the 'Revised European/ American Lymphoma' (REAL) classification for NHL and the WHO. It represents a diffuse tumor with a rich background of lymphocytes with very few Sternberg–Reed cells. It overlaps the diffuse form of lymphocyte predominant sub-variety, the cellular phase of nodular sclerosis and mixed cellularity. The immunological, genetic and clinical features are similar to nodular sclerosis and mixed cellularity varieties.

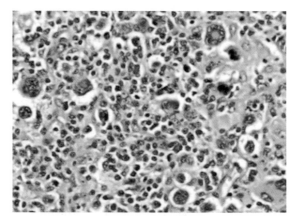

Figure 4.28   A section of a lymph node from a patient with Hodgkin lymphoma, mixed cellularity subtype showing abundant Sternberg–Reed cells (courtesy of Dr Theresa Launders).

Non-Hodgkin lymphoma (NHL)

Although the global incidence of NHL is increasing, it needs to be qualified in view of the wide variation between countries and the specific types of NHL. Follicular lymphoma, for example, is seen most frequently in the US and is more common in the UK than in other European countries or Asia. T-cell lymphomas occur more frequently in certain parts of Asia and South America and certain exceedingly rare subtypes like angiocentric nasal lymphomas seem to be restricted to some of these areas, like Hong Kong (China). Epidemiological studies from the Middle Eastern countries, in particular Saudi Arabia and Kuwait, suggest a higher prevalence of gastrointestinal tract and other extranodal lymphomas; France and Switzerland also record a high incidence of extranodal lymphoma. This wide geographical variation currently remains unexplained.

The classification of NHL has changed many times, as discussed earlier (Chapter 3). In 1994, a panel of international lymphoma specialists proposed a new classification based on clinical pathological syndromes (in their words, 'real' diseases) rather than simple morphology, the common denominator for the majority of previous classifications. Since the majority of these specialists were from Europe and North America, the classification became known as the 'Revised European/American Lymphoma Classification' (REAL). This system was tested in a large international exercise and, following some modifications, endorsed as the 'World Health Organization Classification' (WHO classification) and shown in Table 3.1 (Chapter 3). We think this classification will be updated when new information, such as DNA microarray studies, becomes available and should then remain with us for the foreseeable future! We will discuss the major and some uncommon but unique subtypes here.

In addition to a firm knowledge of the subtype of lymphoma, the specialist needs to have other information which has been deemed to affect the prognosis of individual patients (known as the International Prognostic Index or IPI). The IPI is a summation of a number of specific adverse prognostic factors, which include age greater than 60 years, Ann Arbor Stage III/IV (discussed in Chapter 5), an elevated serum lactate dehydrogenase, reduced performance status (discussed in Chapter 8), and multiple extranodal sites of involvement by lymphoma. The impact of the IPI score on the survival of two cohorts of patients, one afflicted with follicular lymphoma and the other with large cell lymphoma, is shown in Figure 4.29. There is a lesser degree of variation in the prognosis of low grade NHL. Recently a prognostic index, specifically devised for this cohort, known as the Follicular Lymphoma International Prognostic Index (FLIPI) was introduced. It has proven useful for the assessment of patients with low grade NHL.

Lymphoblastic lymphoma

Lymphoblastic lymphoma is a cancer of the precursor cells of T and B lymphocytes and is intimately related to acute lymphoblastic leukemia, with the

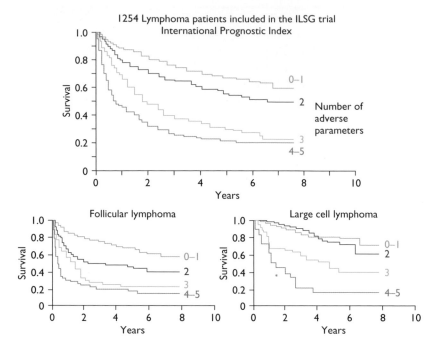

Figure 4.29   The impact of the International Prognostic Index (IPI) on the survival of patients with lymphoma [reproduced with permission from Armitage *et al.* (2003) Lymphomas. *Oxford Textbook of Medicine*, ed Cox *et al.*, Oxford University Press].

principal difference in the mode of its clinical presentation. The distinction is arbitrary and all patients should be treated with an ALL-type treatment. Typically patients with lymphoblastic lymphoma present with lymph node enlargement, usually including the mediastinum (referred to as a mediastinal mass) and will have less than 25% involvement of the bone marrow. Men are affected twice as often as women and the peak age incidence is 15 to 25 years. Most patients have the T-cell variety, but about 10% have the B-cell variety. Central nervous system involvement is common.

Diffuse large B-cell lymphoma

Diffuse large B-cell lymphoma (often simply known as large cell lymphoma) is the most common NHL representing about 35% of all patients (Figure 4.30). Typically it presents *de novo*, but can sometimes arise following the transformation of another lymphoma, such as small lymphocytic, follicular and MALT lymphoma. It usually affects both sexes equally and the median age at diagnosis is about 50 years. It can arise in a nodal (lymphoid) or extranodal site, including unusual sites, such as testis, bone and lung, and tends to have an aggressive biological nature (previously classified as high grade), but is highly responsive to combination chemotherapy with about 40% of patients with advanced-stage disease achieving a cure.

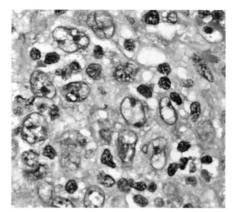

Figure 4.30   A section of a lymph node from a patient with diffuse large B-cell lymphoma showing large lymphoma cells.

Follicular lymphoma

Follicular lymphomas are the second most common type of NHL, accounting for about 30–35% of all lymphomas diagnosed in the US and the UK. They are characterized by an indolent clinical behavior (previously classified as low grade) and the incidence appears to increase with age. The median age at diagnosis is about 55 to 60 years and the majority of patients present with advanced disease. The natural history of follicular lymphoma involves a reduction in the degree of follicularity in the tumor and an increase in the proportion of large cells, with an imminent transformation to a large cell lymphoma. Considerable clinical heterogeneity is characteristic of follicular lymphomas.

Mucosa-associated lymphoid tissue (MALT) lymphoma

MALT lymphomas always present in extranodal sites, in particular eyes (orbital), lungs and stomach. Those arising from the stomach have a well-recognized association with infection by *Helicobacter pylori* (discussed in Chapter 3) and in the early stages can be cured simply by eradication of the infection. They are often associated with cytogenetic abnormalities including trisomy 3 and t(11;18). Sometimes, in particular in the case of thyroid MALT lymphomas and orbital MALT lymphomas, a variety of autoimmune phenomena are recognized, such as Hashimoto's thyroiditis and Sjögren's syndrome. MALT lymphomas can undergo transformation to large cell lymphoma. MALT lymphomas have a slight female predominance with a median age at diagnosis of about 60 years. They often tend to be localized at diagnosis and most patients can be cured at that stage.

Mantle cell lymphoma

Mantle cell lymphoma accounts for about 5 to 8% of all lymphomas and is recognized as a specific entity by virtue of a characteristic cytogenetic abnormality, t(11;14), which involves the BCL-1 gene on chromosome 11 such that the mantle cells overexpress the Bcl-1 protein (also known as cyclin-D). This can be useful in diagnosis, in particular since this lymphoma can have morphological resemblance to small lymphocytic lymphoma, follicular lymphoma and lymphoblastic lymphoma. There is marked male predominance and most patients have advanced disease at diagnosis. In general they tend to have a poor outcome, with most patients faring poorly with conventional treatment.

Burkitt's lymphoma

The hallmark of Burkitt's lymphoma (BL) is the overexpression of the onco-gene *MYC*, resulting from t(8;14), t(2;8), or t(8;22) (Figures 4.14 and 4.15). Three different clinical variants have been described – endemic, sporadic and immunodeficiency BL. The endemic form is usually observed in Africa (in particular equatorial regions) and frequently involves the jaw and kidneys in children aged 4 to 7 years (Figure 3.8); the term 'endemic' was used since the distribution of this BL corresponded to the distribution of endemic malaria. The sporadic variety accounts for about 2% of all adult lymphomas, is typically seen in the US and Western Europe and often presents with a rapidly enlarging abdominal mass. The immunodeficiency variety is frequently observed in patients who are HIV positive. The lymph node section from a patient with Burkitt's lymphoma has a characteristic 'starry sky' appearance (Figure 4.31). All varieties of this lymphoma/leukemia can be cured, in most cases by prompt treatment with intensive chemotherapy in a specialist unit, which we will discuss in Chapter 8.

Peripheral T-cell lymphoma

Peripheral T-cell lymphomas account for about 10 to 15% of all NHL. The accurate diagnosis of peripheral T-cell lymphoma involves a review by an expert hematopathologist and adequate immunological tests. These requirements cannot be stressed enough since the differential diagnosis can be

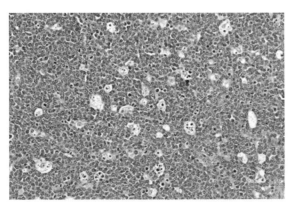

Figure 4.31   A section of a lymph node from a patient with Burkitt's lymphoma; note the 'starry sky' resemblance.

diverse, ranging from a 'benign' T-cell hyperplasia related, for example to a drug reaction or a viral infection, to a diffuse large cell lymphoma. They affect both males and females almost equally and the median age at diagnosis is about 65 years. Most patients present with widespread disease and in general fare poorly.

Anaplastic large T/null-cell lymphoma

Patients with anaplastic lymphoma were often in the past misdiagnosed as having an unrelated cancer, such as an undifferentiated carcinoma. The discovery of the Ki-1 antigen (also known as CD30) led to the recognition of this rare lymphoma. Subsequent discovery of the cytogenetic translocation t(2;5) and the identification of the overexpressed ALK gene led to the confirmation of anaplastic large T/null-cell lymphoma as a separate entity. The median age at diagnosis is 30 years and over 70% of all patients are male. It is crucial to recognize that despite the 'anaplastic' appearance of the lymphoma (Figure 4.32) and frequent poor prognostic features, many patients fare very well with treatment.

Mycosis fungoides/Sézary syndrome

Mycosis fungoides or cutaneous T-cell lymphoma is an indolent lymphoma which arises from T lymphocytes and predominantly involves the skin. It typically presents with a variety of skin disorders, such as eczema and dermatitis, for many years; this phase of the illness is also referred to as the 'erythrodermic' phase. The lesions first manifest themselves superficially but later ulcerate (Figure 4.33). The natural history of mycosis fungoides is to involve the lymph nodes and other organs. Occasionally circulating atypical T lymphocytes with a rather peculiar appearance, and synonymous with T-chronic lymphocytic leukemia, are seen. The disease then resembles leukemia and is known as the leukemic phase of mycosis fungoides, also

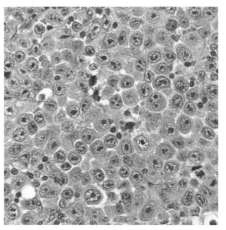

Figure 4.32   A section of a lymph node from a patient with anaplastic lymphoma; note the rather 'aggressive'-looking impression.

77

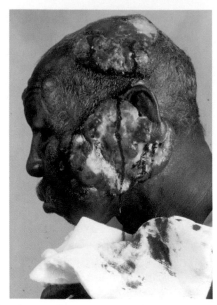

Figure 4.33   Skin lesions in a patient with mycosis fungoides.

termed Sézary syndrome, after Albert Sézary and Yves Bouvrain who described it in Paris in 1938. Sézary syndrome is also sometimes referred to as Baccaredda–Sézary syndrome.

Primary cerebral lymphoma

Primary cerebral lymphoma accounts for 1% of all NHL, but its incidence appears to be rising. It is frequently seen in patients with HIV infection and those who have a compromised immune system from other causes, including recipients of stem cell and other transplants. The patients very rarely have evidence of systemic disease. The presentation is similar to that of a progressively enlarging brain tumor with neurological abnormalities. The imaging studies, such as CT scans and Magnetic Resonance Image (MRI) may suggest unifocal or multifocal disease and the cerebrospinal fluid often reveals atypical lymphocytes. It tends to affect younger patients in general.

Myelomas

Myelomas are characterized by the malignant proliferation of a single clone of plasma cells in the bone marrow producing a paraprotein. They are part of the different conditions resulting in paraproteins, ranging from malignant disorders, like multiple myeloma, Waldenström's macroglobulinemia, plasma cell leukemia and plasmacytomas to benign conditions, such as 'monoclonal gammopathy of undetermined significance' (MGUS), POEMS syndrome (see below) and primary amyloidosis (see Table 3.1).

Multiple myeloma

There are four subtypes of multiple myeloma (typically referred to as simply myeloma or plasma cell myeloma; also known as myelomatosis) dependent on the type of monoclonal protein produced: IgG, IgA, IgD and IgE; IgM is typically associated with Waldenström's macroglobulinemia (see below). The most common is IgG and the rarest is IgE. Each type appears to be associated with a different disease pattern, for example IgA myeloma is associated with more organ damage, such as in the kidneys, than bone disease. About 50% of patients with myeloma have a cytogenetic abnormality, typically involving chromosome 14 (which contains the heavy chain immunoglobulin gene) and deletions of chromosome 13. An important early event in myeloma is the dysregulation of a protein, cyclin D. Rarely a variant of myeloma, called *smoldering myeloma* is diagnosed when the plasma cells in the bone marrow are >10% but <30% and no other findings of myeloma are present.

Monoclonal gammopathy of undetermined significance (MGUS)

MGUS is a condition where a patient is noted by chance to have a paraprotein in the serum but no other features to suggest myeloma. Typically they will have less than 10% plasma cells in the bone marrow, no skeletal lesions, and normal hemoglobin and renal function. Although many of these patients will remain stable, long-term follow-up has shown that about 1% per annum will transform to myeloma. The incidence of both MGUS and myeloma increases with age and the association between these two pathologies supports the notion that most cancers arise as a result of a multi-step (multi-hit) process, with the first oncogenic event causing MGUS and further events leading to myeloma. The recent observation that deletions of chromosome 13 are extremely rare in MGUS, in contrast to abnormalities involving chromosome 14, supports this hypothesis and the presence of 13q− could be useful to predict imminent transformation.

Waldenström's macroglobulinemia

This is a variant of myeloma, first described by Jan Waldenström in Uppsala, Sweden in 1961, in which a high concentration of immunoglobulin M (IgM) paraprotein is found. It is also known as lymphoplasmacytic lymphoma. The incidence is about 0.5 per 100,000 of adult population and the median age at diagnosis is about 65 years, with males being affected more often. Bone lesions are extremely rare and the main classic problems relate to plasma hyperviscosity.

A prognostic staging system based on the level of IgM, hemoglobulin concentration and the beta-2-microglobulin is currently being pursued.

Plasma cell leukemia

Plasma cell leukemia is defined as the presence of more than 20% plasma cells in the peripheral blood. It is classified as *de novo* (60% of cases) or as secondary when it represents leukemic transformation of a previously diagnosed myeloma (40% of cases) (Figure 4.34). The former patients often tend to be under the age of 30 years, have a low level of serum paraprotein, none or few skeletal lesions and a much greater incidence of enlarged liver and spleen. It is frequently associated with renal failure. It is an aggressive disease with a short survival.

Plasmacytoma

Plasmacytomas are a monoclonal collection of plasma cells, which can be solitary, often involving the skeleton, and typically no features of myeloma are noted. In a minority of patients, the disease remains localized for long periods, but in up to 50%, evidence of myeloma appears over a 15- to 20-year period, necessitating careful long-term follow-up. In contrast to solitary plasmacytoma of bone, extramedullary plasmacytoma appears to be a truly localized process with a very low risk of transformation to myeloma.

POEMS syndrome

This is a rare syndrome in which a serum paraprotein is associated with peripheral nerve function abnormalities of the sensorimotor variety (polyneuropathy – P), enlargement of organs, in particular the liver (organomegaly – O), hormonal disturbances (endocrinopathy – E), monoclonal gammopathy (M) and skin changes, in particular hyperpigmentation (S). Interestingly the disease occurs more frequently in Japan, where it is known as Crowe–Fukase syndrome (after Crowe, a British physician and Fukase, a Japanese physician). About 50% of cases are associated with myeloma and most of the remainder with a solitary plasmacytoma. The underlying mechanism for these multisystem changes remains unknown at

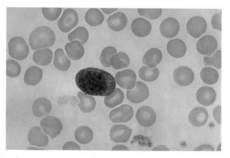

Figure 4.34   A photomicrograph of a blood film from a patient with plasma cell leukemia showing a circulating plasma cell; the absolute plasma cell count is usually more than 2×10^9/liter.

present. It is also known as osteosclerotic myeloma and multicentric Castleman disease.

Primary amyloidosis

Primary amyloidosis (AL), also known as systemic amyloidosis, is a complex multisystem disease that demands astute clinical alertness for prompt diagnosis. Amyloid is a substance consisting of fibrils which contain various proteins that have an ability to acquire more than one conformation, a feature that has earned them the sobriquet of 'chameleon proteins'. In the case of primary amyloidosis, the light chains of the immunoglobulin become crosslinked and are deposited in tissue around the body, in particular in kidney, nerves, liver and heart. In addition almost all patients have serum or urine paraprotein and a monoclonal proliferation of plasma cells in the bone marrow. There are two classes of amyloidosis: in primary amyloidosis the amyloid (AL amyloid) is derived from a clonal proliferation of plasma cells; in contrast, a reactive amyloid or AA amyloid occurs when blood amyloid A protein (an apolipoprotein) is deposited in chronic inflammatory disease, such as rheumatoid arthritis or a chronic infection, such as osteomyelitis. The differentiation of primary amyloidosis from myeloma is arbitrary because both are plasma cell proliferative disorders. The incidence of primary amyloidosis is about 1 per 100,000 adult population and the median age at diagnosis is 64 years.

5 *Diagnosis of leukemia, lymphoma and myeloma*

The way in which blood cancers first show varies and depends to a considerable extent on the precise subtype of disease. Many of the symptoms tend to be non-specific, such as feeling increasingly tired or poorly and it is important to remember that most patients with these symptoms do not have blood cancers. Here we discuss the clinical aspects, including the presentations and how diagnoses are made for leukemias, lymphomas and myelomas.

Leukemia

Initial presentation

Patients with leukemia often present with signs and symptoms arising from bone marrow failure and organ infiltration by the leukemia cells. The symptoms of bone marrow failure include those arising as a result of anemia (too few red cells), infections (too few white blood cells) and bleeding (too few platelets) (Figure 5.1). Anemic people may look pale, may become easily tired

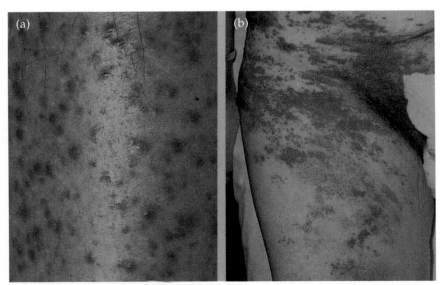

Figure 5.1   (a) A close-up view of bleeding into the skin (petechial hemorrhages) and (b) extensive bleeding (ecchymosis) and bruises over the groin and thigh in a patient with acute myeloid leukemia. (courtesy of Prof Victor Hoffbrand).

83

and, in some cases, may be short of breath. Bone pain and bleeding manifestations are not uncommon. Most patients with acute leukemia give a short history of such symptoms, usually a few weeks to a few months. Acute leukemia rarely presents as an incidental finding on a routine blood test, in contrast to the chronic leukemias. Enlargement of the lymph nodes may occur and organs such as the liver (hepatomegaly) and spleen (splenomegaly) are often affected, in particular in patients with acute lymphoblastic leukemia (ALL) and chronic lymphocytic leukemia (CLL).

Adults with acute myeloid leukemia (AML) often present with non-specific symptoms. However patients with some subtypes of AML present with specific symptoms, for example those with AML subtype M3 usually present with extensive bleeding and sometimes inappropriate thrombosis (clotting). This is due to unique granules within the leukemia cells (see Figure 4.4, Chapter 4), which trigger bleeding and thrombosis (paradoxically) on being released into the bloodstream. Over a third of patients with AML have a serious infection, usually bacterial, at the time of presentation. The most common sites of such infections are chest, bladder, skin and sinuses. The mouth is often involved with a fungal infection (candida or thrush) (Figure 5.2). Fever is the cardinal sign of all infections and in patients with leukemia, other signs of infection may not be present until a later stage. Leukemic infiltration of the skin (called leukemia cutis, Figure 5.3), gums (called gingival hypertrophy, Figure 5.4) and tonsils is often seen in AML subtypes M4 and M5. The spleen is enlarged in about a quarter of all patients with AML.

Patients with ALL, especially children who account for the majority, most commonly present with symptoms of anemia. Alternatively, they may have unprovoked or inappropriate bleeding from unusual places such as gums,

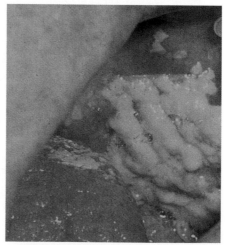

Figure 5.2   Candida (thrush) infection of the buccal mucosa in a patient with lymphocytic leukemia (courtesy of Prof Victor Hoffbrand).

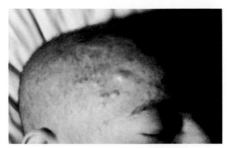

Figure 5.3   Skin involvement (also known as leukemia cutis) in patient with chronic myeloid leukemia in blast crisis.

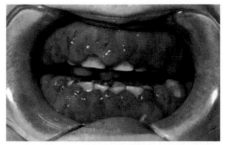

Figure 5.4   Swollen gums (called gingival hypertrophy) in a patient with acute myeloid leukemia of the subtype M5.

intestine or skin, or they become unduly susceptible to infections, developing abscesses or pneumonias, or a fever without an obvious cause (Figure 5.5). Sometimes pain in the arms and legs mimics arthritis or bone infection, in which case leukemia may not be suspected. Rarely patients may present

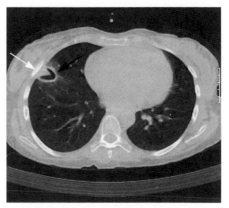

Figure 5.5   A CT scan of a chest showing a fungal infection (arrowed) (in this case, from *Aspergillus flavus*) in a patient with acute lymphoblastic leukemia (courtesy of Prof Victor Hoffbrand).

with respiratory difficulties as a consequence of a mediastinal mass (resulting from lymph nodes swelling) (Figure 5.6).

Occasionally, in both ALL and AML, especially AML subtypes M4 and M5, patients present with central nervous system (CNS) involvement by the leukemia cells. This usually results from infiltration of meninges (lining of the brain), and contamination of the fluid which circulates around the brain and spinal cord (the cerebrospinal fluid or CSF). Rarely the CNS involvement is actually due to the very large number of leukemic cells (called *hyperleukocytosis*) within the brain circulation causing the blood flow to be sluggish. Both ALL and AML can also involve other organs: for example testicular leukemic infiltration is often seen in boys with ALL.

Patients with chronic myeloid leukemia (CML) in the chronic phase (CP) may become tired so gradually, over a period of 3 to 12 months, that they hardly notice the deterioration in their health. They may eventually become short of breath, lose weight or sweat excessively. If the spleen becomes large enough, patients will notice it as a swelling in their abdomen (Figure 5.7). Because of the slow onset of the disease, about a third to a half of all patients with CML are diagnosed following a blood test performed for another purpose, such as before elective surgery, in the antenatal clinic or during routine medical examination. About 1% of males present with a painful erect penis that does not subside (*priapism*). This rare and sometimes embarrassing problem is usually preceded by a short history, of days to a few weeks, of less troublesome intermittent but prolonged penile erections. Over 80% of CML patients will have some splenic enlargement and in about 20% the greatly enlarged spleen may occupy over half of the abdominal cavity.

Patients with CML in the advanced phases tend to present like patients with acute leukemia. Typically the chronic phase (CP) lasts 3 to 6 years but its duration may be shorter or occasionally very much longer. The disease then spontaneously progresses to blast transformation with about 70 to 80% of patients entering a myeloid blast transformation (resembling AML) and the

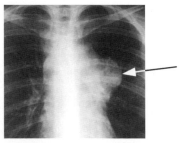

Figure 5.6   Chest radiograph showing a large mediastinal mass (lymph nodes swelling) in a patient with Hodgkin lymphoma (courtesy of Dr John Baird).

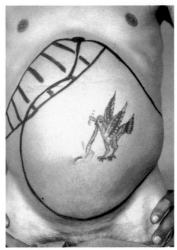

Figure 5.7   Marked splenic enlargement (splenomegaly) in a patient with chronic myeloid leukemia (and a unique sense of humor!).

remainder entering a lymphoid blast transformation (resembling ALL). About half of the patients in the CP transform directly into blast transformation and the rest do so following a period of accelerated phase, with their disease slowly becoming 'aggressive'.

About 40% of all patients with chronic lymphocytic leukemia (CLL) are diagnosed by a routine blood test for unrelated reasons, although they may develop general symptoms such as loss of appetite, loss of weight or undue sweating, especially at night. Alternatively, localized symptoms such as enlarged lymph nodes in the side of the neck, under the arms or in the groin, or an enlarged spleen may alert them to the problem (Figure 5.8). Some patients with CLL have increased susceptibility to infections, especially bacterial, and will often present with chest or bladder infections; they can also develop viral infections such as herpes zoster (shingles) (Figure 5.9). In due course, as the disease progresses, most patients develop infections.

Diagnosis

The diagnosis of leukemia may be suspected from automated analysis of blood taken from a vein in the arm. Normally the number of white blood cells in the blood ranges from 3.5 to 10×10^9/liter. Patients with leukemia frequently, though not always, have increased white blood cells, usually in the range of 20 to 200×10^9/liter. This is the finding which usually attracts the doctor's attention. Importantly, there are many other causes for a moderatedly raised white blood cell count (up to about 20×10^9/liter), such as bacterial infections, but very high levels are likely due to leukemia.

87

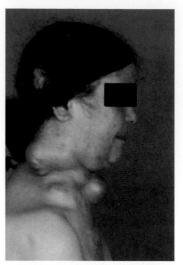

Figure 5.8   Marked neck lymph node enlargement in a patient with chronic lymphocytic leukemia.

The next step is to examine the blood under a microscope. Although special stains are used to enable the various types of cell to be identified, it is not always possible to tell which type of white blood cell predominates. However, if most of the white blood cells are of the immature variety (blast cells), then the diagnosis of acute leukemia is highly likely. In most cases it is possible to distinguish AML from ALL by examining the patient's blood, although occasionally the distinction is difficult and further tests are required (Figure 5.10). A diagnosis of CML or CLL is often straightforward when the white blood cell count is over 50×10^9/liter.

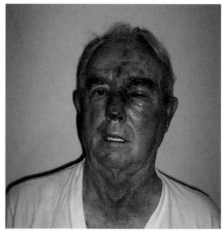

Figure 5.9   Shingles (*Herpes zoster*) infection involving the left side of the face in a patient with chronic lymphocytic leukemia.

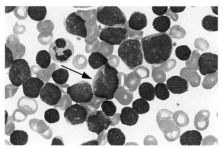

Figure 5.10   A photomicrograph of blast cells (arrowed) from a patient suffering from acute undifferentiated leukemia (neither AML, nor ALL).

Occasionally the white blood cell count is normal or even low, and other blood abnormalities might indicate the presence of leukemia. In such cases, examination of the bone marrow is necessary. In practice, examination of the marrow is carried out routinely in all newly diagnosed patients, even when the diagnosis has already been established by blood examination, because it gives a great deal of extra information that is necessary in planning the treatment.

Marrow examination is relatively simple and can be obtained by needle aspiration, percutaneous trephine biopsy or surgical biopsy. The usual methods are needle aspiration/percutaneous trephine biopsy. The procedure typically does not require sedation and the doctor, physician assistant or a specialist nurse anesthetizes the skin over the hip bone (iliac crest) and inserts a medical needle (such as a Jamshidi needle, or similar) until it touches the bone (see Figure 5.11); sometimes a needle aspiration is performed by puncture of the sternum (breast bone). The needle is then gradually advanced through the thick layer of outer bone and into the spongy cavity that contains the marrow (also known as red marrow). A syringe attached to the needle is used

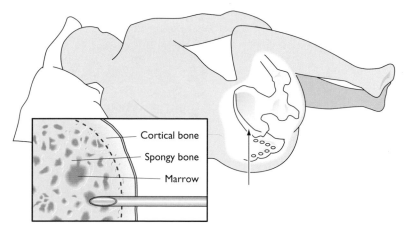

Figure 5.11   Schematic representation of a bone marrow procedure.

to suck out about 3 to 5 milliliters of marrow cells mixed with blood and thereafter a micro-biopsy (about 2 mm bore) is obtained. In very young children, the samples are usually obtained from the upper end of the tibia (the large bone in the lower part of the leg, between the knee and the ankle). The samples are then stained (to bring out details) and examined under a microscope. Marrow aspirate sample allows the assessment of all stages of hemopoiesis and the trephine biopsy provides a core of bone and bone marrow to show architecture.

The marrow of patients with acute leukemia is densely packed with cells, most of them blast cells (Figure 5.12). This is very different from the appearance of normal marrow, in which cells of many different shapes and sizes are seen in different proportions. Marrow packed with blast cells is occasionally found even when no blast cells are found in the patient's blood. The marrow of patients with chronic leukemia is similar to that seen in acute leukemia in that it is densely packed with cells, but in CML these cells are granulocytes in all stages of maturation, similar to those seen in the blood. In CLL, the cells normally present in the marrow are replaced to varying degrees by small lymphocytes similar to those found in excess in the blood. The proportion of lymphocytes in the marrow may range from 40% to over 90%.

It is customary to carry out a battery of specialized tests on the marrow and blood cells to establish the identity and the presence (or absence) of various immunological markers on the leukemic cell surface or inside the cell. Most specialist laboratories use a panel of monoclonal antibodies which enable the specialist to determine the nature of the leukemic cells. These reagents are usually used with automated techniques, such as flow cytometry, which have considerable advantages over traditional microscopy, particularly the speed and accurate quantitative assessment of the cells. This latter feature is particularly useful in monitoring patients following treatment.

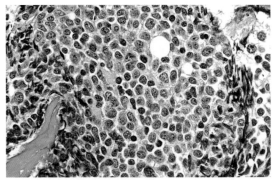

Figure 5.12   A photomicrograph of bone marrow from a patient with acute lymphoid leukemia (in this case, pre-B ALL) showing complete replacement by lymphoblasts.

Many other tests are available to help the specialist characterize the leukemic cells more precisely, to provide information that may be useful in planning the treatment, and for research purposes (any test conducted purely for research does, of course, require the patient's informed consent). For example tests can be performed to determine which of a number of possible enzymes are present in the cytoplasm of the leukemic cells, and whether or not certain marker proteins produced only by the leukemic cells, such as ZAP 70 in the case of CLL, are present in the cell surface.

A particularly valuable test is to examine the chromosomal make-up of the leukemic cells (discussed in Chapter 3). Loss or gain of whole chromosomes, chromosome breaks and loss, inversion or translocation of a part of a chromosome can be detected. Most laboratories now offer a particularly sensitive technique, known as *fluorescence* in situ *hybridization* or FISH, for detecting chromosomal abnormalities (Figure 5.13). In AML, for instance, the presence

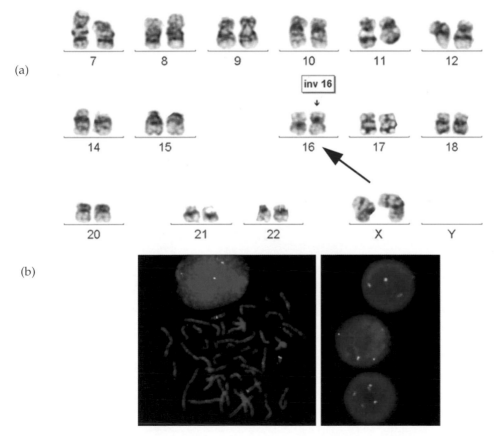

Figure 5.13   Photomicrographs of two cytogenetic abnormalities often associated with a good prognosis in acute myeloid leukemia: (a) an inversion of chromosome 16 (arrowed) and (b) + (8;21); red (chromosome 8), green (chromosome 21).

of a t(8;21) translocation or a chromosome 16 inversion identifies patients with good prognosis, whereas the t(9;22) translocation in ALL is associated with a poor outcome. Chromosomal translocations are also used to identify patients who will benefit from intensifying the dose of chemotherapy and even to select the best drugs. We will discuss these aspects further in Chapter 8.

An increasing number of specialist laboratories are using DNA-based techniques to help the specialist identify the precise genes afflicted and to characterize the leukemia accordingly. This important technology, called 'gene microarray profiling' (or simply microarray) determines the level of expression of thousands of genes simultaneously and the information can then be used to establish the prognosis with a much higher degree of accuracy (Figure 5.14). It has recently been established that there are several molecularly distinct hematological cancers within the same morphological

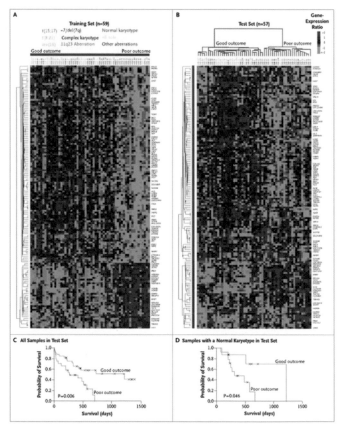

Figure 5.14   DNA microarray analysis from patients with acute myeloid leukemia [reproduced with permission from Bullinger *et al.* (2004) Use of gene-expression profiling to identify prognostic subclasses in adult myeloid leukemia, *N Engl J Med* 350: 1605–16].

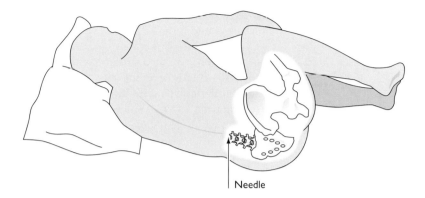

Needle

Figure 5.15   Schematic representation of a spinal tap (lumbar puncture).

category, so clearly microarray tests should prove most useful and (hopefully) allow us to tailor appropriate treatment accordingly. Should the preliminary results be confirmed, it is possible that microarray tests could substitute for the multiple diagnostic tests which are currently required to collate the relevant prognostic information.

The cerebrospinal fluid (CSF) should be examined for the presence of leukemia cells in all patients with ALL, who have a high risk of central nervous system (CNS) involvement and in all other patients who have neurological abnormalities, for example patients with AML subtype M4 and M5, or CML in blast crisis. In the latter case, it is critical to exclude raised intracranial pressure prior to carrying out a lumbar puncture, by performing appropriate imaging studies. The lumbar puncture, like a bone marrow procedure, is a relatively simple procedure which does not require sedation. It is carried out by inserting a needle into a space between the 4th and the 5th lumbar vertebrae (Figure 5.15).

Lymphomas

Initial presentation

Patients with HL often present with constitutional symptoms, such as weight loss, profuse sweating (especially at night), weakness, fatigue and anorexia. Clinically many of these patients have painless enlargement of lymph nodes, in particular those in the neck. Neck nodes are involved in about 60 to 70% of all patients, followed by involvement of the axillary (armpit) nodes in about 15% of the patients. Other nodes, such as the inguinal (groin) nodes are involved in about 10% of all patients. The nodes often fluctuate in size, and alcohol ingestion may precipitate pain. Splenomegaly is noted in about a third of all patients but it is seldom massive. Enlargement of the liver may also occur. Involvement of sites which are not part of the lymphatic system (called extranodal), such as lung, CNS, skin and bone is uncommon, but may occur.

Patients with NHL can also present with constitutional complaints such as fever, night sweats and weight loss, but the frequency is considerably less than that seen in patients with Hodgkin lymphoma. The majority of patients have asymmetric painless enlargement of lymph nodes in one or more peripheral lymph node regions, such as neck and axillary or groin. The liver and spleen are enlarged in about a quarter of all patients. Extranodal disease is more common in NHL than in HL, and sites which are often affected include the stomach, brain, skin, testes, eyes and thyroid gland.

Although lymphoma is clinically heterogeneous, various clinical patterns have been noted for the different subtypes. The low-grade lymphomas, such as follicular lymphoma (Figure 5.16) and small lymphocytic lymphoma, often tend to have an indolent clinical behavior, are more common in patients over the age of 60 years, are often widely disseminated at presentation with generalized lymph node enlargement, which can be gradual or intermittent and patients may have few constitutional symptoms. Other indolent lymphomas, such as splenic marginal zone lymphoma, present almost exclusively with a large spleen. Variants include extranodal marginal zone lymphoma (previously known as maltoma) which presents with symptoms related to affected sites. For example the gastric variety, which is often associated with infection by *Helicobacter pylori*, presents with abdominal discomfort, feeling bloated and heartburn. Cutaneous lymphomas, such as mycosis fungoides, affect the skin and present with widespread psoriatic-like lesions which progress to plaque and tumor formation over long periods of time, sometimes several years, but in the later stages affect lymph nodes, other organs and blood (such as in Sézary syndrome) (Figure 5.17).

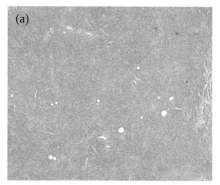
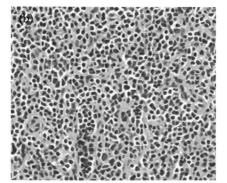

Figure 5.16   A lymph node section from a patient with a low-grade follicular lymphoma. (a) low and (b) high magnification showing a clonal population of B lymphocytes.

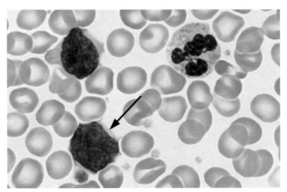

Figure 5.17   A photomicrograph of a Sézary lymphoma cell (arrowed).

Patients with high-grade lymphomas, such as diffuse large B-cell lymphoma, typically present with a short history of rapidly enlarging lymph nodes and often with constitutional symptoms. Extranodal sites are frequently involved (Figure 5.18). Rarely patients afflicted with some of the other varieties of high-grade lymphomas, such as Burkitt's lymphoma, present in a unique manner. For instance, most patients with Burkitt's lymphoma in the UK and US present with abdominal complaints, such as pain and distension, in contrast to African patients with Burkitt's lymphoma who present with jaw tumors. HIV-related lymphomas are usually aggressive and frequently present with CNS disease. Likewise, those afflicted with other specific varieties, such as testicular and other extranodal lymphomas, present uniquely. Those with testicular NHL typically present with a testicular swelling, and those with extranodal NHL with symptoms pertinent to the primary organ involvement, for example, stomach NHL presents with gastric complaints such as abdominal discomfort, bloatedness and anorexia. Rarely patients with CNS lymphoma present with symptoms of headaches, blurred vision, weakness and speech difficulties.

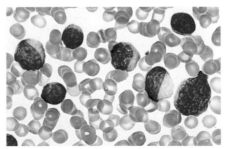

Figure 5.18   Peripheral blood film showing lymphoma cells from a patient who presented with pancytopenia.

Diagnosis

The diagnosis of all lymphomas is typically made by histological examination of an excised lymph node. Both HL and NHL have distinctive morphological signatures which allow for the specific diagnosis to be made in the majority of cases. In a minority, the distinction between these two entities can prove difficult and specialized tests, such as the microarray tests (discussed above) can be useful.

Blood and bone marrow examination is important in the evaluation of all lymphoma patients. Bone marrow involvement is common in low-grade lymphomas and sometimes lymphoma cells may be seen in the blood also. Anemia is common in both HL and NHL and does not necessarily indicate marrow involvement. In patients with extensive marrow involvement, the blood counts are often decreased (pancytopenia). A variety of blood biochemical abnormalities, such as high levels of uric acid and calcium, can be present and dictate that a comprehensive biochemical profile be part of the assessment. Elevated levels of the enzyme lactate dehydrogenase (LDH) have an important prognostic significance and in the case of NHL are a part of the International Prognostic Index.

Imaging investigations are mandatory and currently all patients with lymphoma have computed tomography (CT) scans of the thorax (chest), abdomen and pelvis (Figure 5.19). Imaging with radio isotopic bone scans, skeletal X-rays, or magnetic resonance imaging (MRI) will be indicated for specific clinical reasons, for example if CNS or bone involvement is suspected. Recently positron emission tomography (PET) scans (Figure 5.20), which exploit the abnormal glucose metabolism in cancer cells and are, therefore, functional rather than anatomical, have entered the clinic. Studies have confirmed their usefulness in confirming recurrence and predicting response to treatment in some cases of lymphomas. Currently, however, PET scans alone might not provide enough information and, if available, should be used along with CT or MRI.

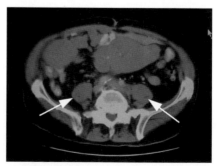

Figure 5.19   A CT scan of the abdomen in a patient with Burkitt's lymphoma showing multiple enlarged lymph glands (arrowed) (courtesy of Dr John Baird).

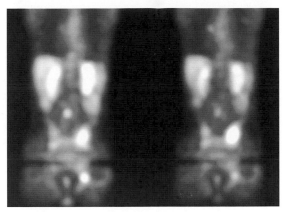

Figure 5.20   A PET scan showing lymph node enlargement in a patient with Hodgkin lymphoma.

Other specialized tests, such as endoscopy, will be required for specific presentations, for example if a gastric lymphoma is suspected. In patients suspected to have CNS disease and in those with a subtype of lymphoma associated with a high risk of CNS involvement, for example lymphoblastic lymphoma and Burkitt's lymphoma, a lumbar puncture will be performed.

Clinical staging is mandatory for most patients with lymphomas. It defines the extent and distribution of the disease in the individual patient and has important treatment and prognostic relevance. Currently the staging systems are anatomical and with increasing use of PET scans and molecular diagnostic tools, we can anticipate significant revisions to be made in the near future. For patients with lymphomas, both HL and NHL, a clinical staging system, such as the one depicted in Table 5.1, is useful.

Table 5.1 The clinical staging system for lymphomas	
Stage I	Involvement of a single lymph node region or lymphoid structure (e.g. spleen)
Stage II	Involvement of two or more lymph node regions on the same side of the diaphragm
Stage III	Involvement of lymph node regions or structures on both sides of the diaphragm
Stage IV	Disseminated disease involving one or more extranodal site(s) beyond that designated the suffix 'E'
The suffix 'A' is added to designate an absence of 'B' symptoms; the suffix 'B' is added if the patient has fever, drenching sweats or weight loss; the suffix 'E' designates involvement of a single extranodal site; the suffix 'X' implies 'bulky' disease.	

In the 1970s, some patients with HL were subjected to abdominal exploratory surgery (laparotomy), often accompanied by removal of the spleen (for histologic examination). With the changing therapeutic approaches, in particular for early-stage Hodgkin lymphoma, and the high quality of CT scans, laparotomy and splenectomy are no longer performed as part of the routine staging. Laproscopy (key-hole exploration of the abdomen) may occasionally be required for diagnostic purposes in all lymphomas. Another historical investigation, a lymphogram, which used to be the preferred method to study the abdominal lymph nodes, is now rarely offered because it is very time-consuming and less informative than CT scans.

Many efforts are being directed to the molecular diagnosis of lymphomas also. Gene microarray tests have confirmed that within certain subtypes, for example diffuse large B-cell lymphoma, there are at least three distinct signatures, suggesting that there are different subgroups within this subtype. It is of note that this clinical distinction was evident even after the patients were classified according to the International Prognostic Index and, therefore, has important prognostic relevance and should lead to better stratification of patients for appropriate treatments (Figure 5.21). Similar efforts were very recently reported in patients with follicular lymphoma, which has a widely variable clinical course. Interestingly, in follicular lymphomas the genes that best defined prognosis were expressed in the microenvironment (such as T cells, macrophages and dendritic cells), but not the follicular lymphoma cells themselves. This clearly differentiates follicular lymphoma from, for example, diffuse large B-cell lymphoma, in which the prognostic signatures are based on genes expressed by the lymphoma cells. We will discuss these aspects further in Chapter 8.

Myelomas

Initial presentation

Most patients with myeloma present with bone pain and symptoms of anemia. The most frequent sites of pain are the back and the rib cage and some patients may have fractures (called pathological since they usually arise in the absence of trauma). The anemia is often mild and arises gradually. About a third of all patients will also show signs of renal (kidney) problems, though these are severe in less than 5%. This is commonly due to myeloma proteins damaging the kidneys (called 'myeloma' kidney), but other factors, for example infections, high calcium and amyloid deposition, may contribute. Repeated infections are often a problem and arise as a result of the lack of a normal immune system (normal immunoglobulins are lacking – *immunoparesis*) and in the advanced stages, low neutrophil counts (as a result of increasing marrow infiltration). Some patients may have abnormal bleeding as the myeloma proteins may interfere with platelet function and coagulation factors; in advanced stages, low platelet counts may occur.

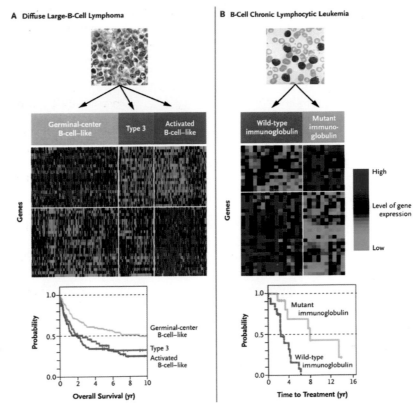

Figure 5.21   Examples of molecularly and clinically distinct subgroups of lymphoma (Panel A) and leukemia (Panel B). [reproduced with permission from Staudt LM (2003) Molecular diagnosis of the hematologic cancers, *N Engl J Med* 348: 1777–85].

Rarely the very high levels of myeloma proteins, in particular the subtypes IgA and IgM, may result in increasing the viscosity of the blood and cause impairment of the CNS function, which requires urgent treatment. Deposition of the amyloid protein occurs in about 10% of myeloma patients. This can lead to a variety of serious problems, in addition to the kidney problems discussed above. It can cause damage to the nerves (peripheral neuropathy), heart (by damaging the heart muscle), muscles, skin and joints. Very seldomly it can result in thickening of the tongue (*macroglossia*) and a diarrheal syndrome by involving the bowel (Figure 5.22).

Rarely spinal cord compression or nerve root compression can occur as a direct result of a collection of myeloma cells (plasmacytoma) (Figure 5.23a and b); very rarely such a collection of myeloma cells can result in swellings in most unusual places, such as the back of the eyes (Figure 5.24).

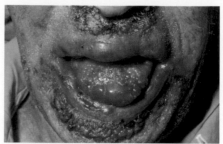

Figure 5.22   Thickening of the tongue and lips due to nodules and waxy deposits of amyloid in a patient with myeloma (courtesy of Prof Victor Hoffbrand).

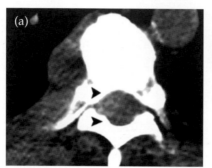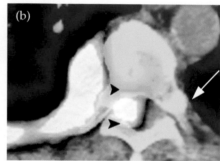

Figure 5.23   A CT scan (a) and a PET-CT scan (b) showing spinal cord compression in a patient with a plasmacytoma (arrowed) (Courtesy of Dr John Baird).

About a quarter of myeloma patients are diagnosed as a result of being found to have abnormal blood tests on routine screening, or being investigated for an unrelated problem. Patients affected with some of the rare subtypes, such as Waldenström's macroglobulinemia, typically present with enlarged lymph nodes and a large spleen; bony disease is uncommon. Jan Waldenström described hyperviscosity in association with this disorder over 50 years ago.

Diagnosis

Nearly all patients with myeloma have an abnormal protein, known as myeloma protein (M protein), in the blood or urine, or both. This is detected by a technique called protein electrophoresis (Figure 5.25). Most laboratories use a technique called immunofixation to enhance the results of 'standard' protein electrophoresis. Immunofixation gives more rapid results than standard protein electrophoresis, and it is more sensitive. In most patients this is of the subtype IgG, followed by IgA, with rare cases of IgM; IgD and IgE are very rare. It is important to note that many diseases are associated with M

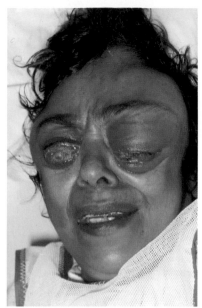

Figure 5.24   Bilateral swellings occurring behind the eyes (orbital) in a patient with myeloma.

proteins. These include benign causes, such as monoclonal gammopathy, also known as MGUS. It is, however, important to monitor all patients with M proteins for a progressive rise, which may herald the emergence of myeloma. Rarely it is associated with other cancers arising from the lymphatic system, such as CLL and lymphomas. Typically the levels of the M protein are the highest in patients with myeloma. The increased protein can cause a unique phenomenon in the blood, whereby the red cells appear to be stacked like coins (*rouleaux*) (Figure 5.26).

Other biochemical investigations of prognostic relevance, other than kidney function tests, include a test for a protein called beta-2-microglobulin, which is often raised and higher levels correlate with worse prognosis. The blood calcium and albumin levels also carry a prognostic relevance. The blood usually confirms the presence of anemia and a test known as erythrocyte sedimentation rate or ESR is typically high in myeloma patients.

A bone marrow examination is an essential diagnostic investigation. Typically the marrow shows increased plasma cells, often with abnormal forms (myeloma cells) (Figure 5.27). Rarely myeloma cells account for over 70% of all marrow cells and if an examination of the blood confirms large numbers of similar cells (usually more than 2×10^9 myeloma cells per liter), then the diagnosis of a plasma cell leukemia is preferred. In advanced myeloma, it is not uncommon to see a few circulating myeloma cells in the

101

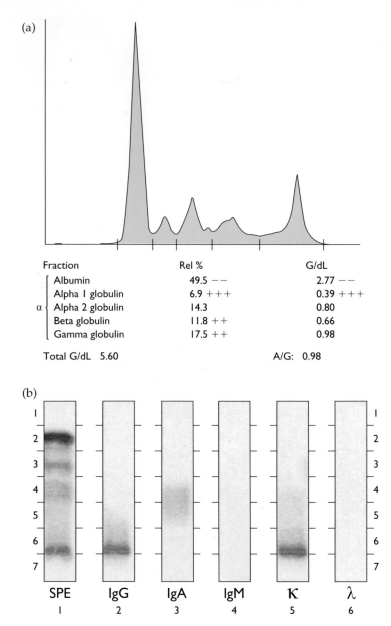

Figure 5.25   Serum protein electrophoresis (SPE) carried out on a blood specimen from a patient with an IgGκ myeloma, (a) an abnormal spike and (b) a gel representation.

blood. Special stains are useful to confirm the diagnosis when there is a modest increase in the myeloma cells. Cytogenetic analysis on the marrow cells is carried out, in particular to detect the presence (or absence) of the chromosome 13q− abnormality, which carries a graver prognosis.

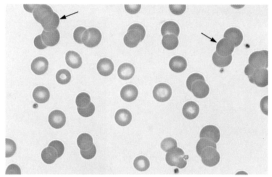

Figure 5.26   *Rouleaux* formation of red blood cells (arrowed) in a patient with myeloma.

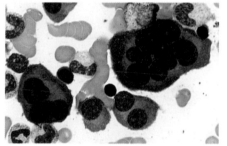

Figure 5.27   Specimen of bone marrow from a patient with myeloma showing multinucleated and binucleated plasma cells.

A skeletal survey (also known as a myeloma scan) should be performed in all patients. This survey usually includes radiography of the entire spine, skull, chest, pelvic, both humeri (upper arm) and both femora (thighs). Typically a combination of osteoporosis, lytic lesions and fractures is seen (Figures 5.28 and 5.29). MRI scans are also very useful in providing additional information, since they can visualize the marrow directly (but not the cortical bone). MRIs are also useful in the follow-up of patients at high risk of developing myeloma, such as those with MGUS, plasmacytoma and smoldering myeloma. PET scans might also prove useful for such situations.

Confirmation of the diagnosis of myeloma is usually based on the finding of M protein, bone marrow infiltration by myeloma cells and the presence of lytic lesions on radiography. The principal differential diagnosis in a patient with M protein but without other features of myeloma is MGUS. The currently accepted diagnostic criteria for myeloma are shown in Table 5.2, but not all cases fulfil these criteria.

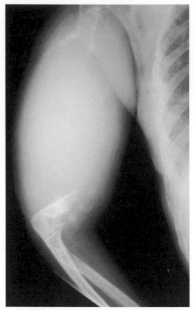

Figure 5.28   Radiograph of the right upper arm from a patient with myeloma showing almost complete destruction of the humerus bone.

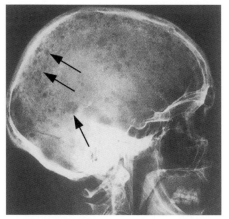

Figure 5.29   Skull radiograph from a patient with myeloma showing numerous lytic lesions (arrowed).

| Table 5.2 |
| Diagnostic criteria for multiple myeloma |

A. Major criteria: (1) Increased plasma cells in the bone marrow (>30%)

(2) Paraprotein in serum (IgG >3.5 g/dL; IgA >2 g/dL) and/or urine
    (> 1 g/24 h of Bence-Jones protein)

(3) Plasmacytoma on biopsy

B. Minor criteria: (1) Increased plasma cells in the bone marrow (10–30%)

(2) Paraprotein present, but less than (2) above

(3) Lytic bone lesions

(4) Reduced normal immunoglobulins (<50% normal)

A diagnosis of multiple myeloma requires a minimum of one major and one minor criteria or three minor criteria which must include (1) and (2), but not all cases fulfill these criteria. Other factors, such as the presence of a myeloma kidney, are important additional factors which need to be taken into account.

| Table 5.3 |
| The Durie–Salmon staging system for multiple myeloma |

	Stage I	Stage II	Stage III
Tumor cell mass	Low All of the following:	Medium Not fitting stage I or III	High
Monoclonal IgG (g/L)	<50		>70
Monoclonal IgA (g/L)	<30		>50
Bence-Jones protein excretion	<4		>12
Hb (g/dL)	>10		<8.5
Calcium (mmol/L)	<2.6		>2.6
Lytic lesions	None or 1		More than 1

The suffix 'A' is added for serum creatinine <175 μmol/L
The suffix 'B' is added for serum creatinine >175 μmol/L

Following the establishment of the diagnosis of myeloma, it is useful to stage the individual patients, as the outlook depends on this. The Durie–Salmon staging system, introduced in 1975 and based on a number of clinical and laboratory parameters, remains the most widely used system (see Table 5.3). It reflects the overall myeloma burden and behavior, but does not include some of the more recently recognized prognostic factors, such as the abnormal chromosome 13 or the blood beta-2-microglobulin and albumin levels. Undoubtedly a revised staging system should follow soon, particularly as more sophisticated analysis of myeloma molecular biology is applied.

A diagnosis of amyloidosis is made by biopsy of tongue, gums, abdominal fat or rectum with special staining (called Congo red) for the amyloid protein. Specialized tests are sometimes necessary to establish if the amyloid is AL (primary) or AA (reactive).

6 *The patient and the specialist*

The diagnosis of a blood cancer is often made in a roundabout way. Initially a patient may be referred from one hospital/clinic to another, before he or she receives any real explanation. The news usually comes as a (psychological) bombshell to both the patient and his or her relatives, and, perhaps, as a surprise to the family physician. Most patients are deeply upset and may even be resentful. If they feel that the diagnosis was delayed for some time, they may wonder whether their chances of being cured have been jeopardized. Some patients will be annoyed to see most, if not all, previously performed tests repeated at the specialized center. Naturally most patients and their relatives may feel despondent.

The patients will wonder why it happened to them; they may feel guilt that the disease results from something they have done or could have avoided doing. Parents may ask 'Why my child?' and wonder if other family members will be affected. The specialist therefore is faced not only with the difficult task of informing the patient and his or her relatives about the diagnosis but also with helping them to cope with the news. The specialist's approach is likely to be guided by the precise type of blood cancer, as well as by the patient's age, clinical condition and ability to understand. Many patients (and parents and relatives) want to know about the causes of their cancers in general and of their own disease in particular. Most specialists will explain the possible roles of environmental factors, such as radiation, toxic chemicals and viruses, but they will also admit that it is almost always impossible to determine the true contribution of such factors in individual cases.

Communication between the patient and the specialist

Communication in the English language is often defined as to 'make known' or 'to impart', but its Latin derivation might be more appropriate in the context of communication between the patient and the specialist. The word 'communicate' is derived from the Latin word *'communis'*, which means 'in common' and although the main aim remains to elicit and impart information, the *modus operandi* in which this exercise is carried out is very important. It can have a profound effect on the present and future relationship between the patient and the specialist, and importantly, on the patient's approach to his or her disease and treatment. Currently there is significant emphasis worldwide in incorporating good communication skills in medical school curricula, compared with just a decade ago, when most schools offered little or no such training. Good communication skills improve diagnostic accuracy, reduce patient anxiety and uncertainty and provide an appropriate infrastructure for the specialised investigations and treatment.

Lesley Fallowfield, from Brighton (UK), and others have repeatedly shown how good communication can lead to better patient compliance and may also be an effective way to minimize medico-legal litigation. Good specialists acknowledge the importance of good, honest communication and recognize the enormous contributions which patients make and respect their individual sensitivities accordingly.

Communicating with the young patient

If a leukemia or a lymphoma is diagnosed in a child, the specialist will probably talk first with the parents or guardians and explain the prognosis and the potential treatment strategy. At this stage, and perhaps also later, the specialist will probably emphasize that statistics relate only imprecisely to individual patients, and that, while there is a very good chance that the child will be cured, the possibility of failure must not be entirely discounted.

Children usually suspect that something serious is wrong with them by the time they and their parents or guardians visit the specialist. How much a specialist chooses to tell a young patient depends very much on the individual circumstances; however, it may be perfectly reasonable to explain to a child that he or she has a disease that may be fatal if appropriate treatment is not given. This should certainly help to emphasize to the child the need to collaborate in the treatment program. Many children appreciate such an approach and might benefit from talking with other young patients. They should be reassured that it is accepted to feel sad and cry, and pretty 'cool' to ask questions. It is also important to urge the child to maintain contact with school and friends.

In many countries it is a legal requirement to provide a child with cancer with information commensurate to their age and understanding. The Children's Act of 1989 in the UK and the United Nations Convention on the Rights of the Child (1989) exhort those involved in the care of children to inform the child of their situation, to solicit their opinion and when appropriate to regard their opinion as binding. Clearly this may seem a huge responsibility for the child. They will look for advocates such as their parents, nursing and medical staff or a social worker to help support them with making decisions regarding their care. This legal precedent was set to facilitate a child's autonomy and to promote a 'smooth' transition to independence in adult life.

Communicating with the adult patient

The vast majority of patients afflicted with leukemias, lymphomas, in particular the high-grade varieties, or myelomas are adults. Even though as recently as two decades ago it was customary in many cultures to conceal the diagnosis from patients and to inform relatives, it is today normal practice, worldwide, to give the newly diagnosed patient details of the diagnosis and, to explain some features about the biology of the disease, the relevant statistics and the treatment that will be used to try and achieve remission and hopefully, cure. In today's medical culture, there is a trend to move away from traditional medical paternalism towards frank information sharing and patient-centered decision making. Many patients have already spent considerable time researching and surfing the internet-fed jungle of medical information (and misinformation) and will be well informed generally and not expect striking revelations about their disease. Despite this (or in spite of this), the most difficult question of all is when the patient asks 'Doctor, how long do I have to live?' It is always impossible to give an accurate answer to this question and therefore the best approach is for the specialist to explain the expected range of survival, such as one patient may die within a few weeks of diagnosis whereas another may eventually be cured. Statistics apply to populations, not individuals, and therefore cannot accurately predict survival for the individual patient.

Leukemias

Most adults with acute leukemia will have AML, but some will have ALL. Many patients with children will be concerned that there may be a risk that it is passed on genetically; however, until we know much more about the causes of leukemia, we can say quite simply that the risk of it occurring twice in one family is only very slightly greater than one would expect from chance alone. Patients are often concerned that a chemical with which they have come into contact may have caused or contributed to their leukemia. In most cases, the specialist is asked about the possible role of a specific chemical; usually, however, it is difficult for the specialist to give an answer because no clear evidence exists one way or the other. However, if a patient is exposed to radiation or benzene or a closely related compound, he or she may well be entitled to compensation from an employer, and legal advice should be sought. Some people are concerned about whether their leukemia (or other cancers) is contagious and they should be reassured that no leukemia can be caught from, or passed on to, another person.

In the case of chronic leukemias, a frank discussion at the time of diagnosis is equally important, even if the patients have absolutely no symptoms. It is useful to draw attention to the fact that chronic means slowly progressive, and the specialist will explain the implications of this. The patient with CML will be told of the different phases of the disease and the unpredictability of the onset of transformation. They will be told of the current, rather contrasting forms of treatments which are best (based on current evidence) for them. When talking to the patient with CLL, the specialist will stress that not every patient requires treatment and some patients live for 20 or more years following diagnosis, though the average is less.

Lymphomas

With the bimodal age incidence of Hodgkin lymphoma, the first peak is in young adults, many of whom are college/university students. There will be a lot of concerns with regards to a possible infectious agent etiology, positive associations with size of families, higher socio-economic status, housing, parental education and family history. Much of this is fueled by the numerous speculations, some initiated by Hodgkin himself in 1832, followed by Sternberg in 1898 and Reed in 1902. The specialist will discuss the current scenario with regard to the only established potential risk factor, which is the Epstein–Barr virus (EBV), based on the finding of EBV DNA in up to 50% of tumor biopsies (chapter 4). The specialist will emphasize that although many patients will be cured, sadly some will die from the disease and a few from the side-effects of the treatment (chapter 10).

Most of the lymphomas afflicting adults under the age of 60 tend to be high grade and most will require treatment. Low-grade lymphomas are usually seen in patients over the age of 60 years and it is important to recognize that not everyone will require treatment; some will be observed carefully and offered treatment only when they are symptomatic or have progressive disease. Many of the low-grade lymphomas have a long natural history, characterized by fluctuating levels of disease activity. The specialist will point out that, like CLL, many patients will live for long periods and some will even attain their natural life expectancy, but will always have the disease.

Myelomas

Since most patients with myeloma cannot be cured at present, the first question that the specialist might address is to ascertain if therapy is required and, if so, what is the best choice of treatment and the specific goals. The specialist will also discuss the importance of monitoring all patients with an elevated myeloma protein who do not fulfil the diagnostic criteria for myeloma. Many patients have concerns about the bony destruction and the associated disability, even when treatment directed against their myeloma is successful. Some patients will have concerns of a possible link of the use of pesticides and hair dyes and their myeloma, largely based on recent media reports. Epidemiological evidence does not suggest a firm causal association. There are some reports of a possible increased incidence of myeloma in persons exposed to benzene and some petroleum refinery products, but as in the case of leukemias, it is almost impossible to incriminate a causal association in individual patients.

Communicating with the older patients

In most cultures, older patients tend to seek less information and are often less involved in the treatment decision-making process. Specialists will be very much aware of this and will often offer 'escape clauses', which allow them to accommodate matters commensurate to the local cultures and the individual's philosophies; for example an older patient in Palm Springs, California may have totally different expectations from the specialist and may well wish to be treated in the same manner as a young(er) adult, whereas an older patient in rural Yorkshire, UK, might well sum up matters by saying 'Doctor, just do what you think is right, spare me the 'gory' details and get on with it'!

Concluding remarks

Finally, specialists recognize that most patients, even the best-informed ones, are stunned by the diagnosis of a blood cancer and in their bewildered state may only comprehend part of the discussions which take place. Most specialists will be very accommodating and encourage patients and their relatives to ask questions; moreover, they will understand that much of what is said initially may need to be repeated later. The specialist may also suggest professional psychosocial support, in addition to a variety of support organizations, such as the Leukemia and Lymphoma Societies in the US and UK, the International Myeloma Foundation in the US, UK and Germany, the global José Carreras Foundation and other reputable worldwide organizations. For the convenience of the reader (and the patient), some of the worldwide support organizations, with appropriate means of contact, are listed in Appendix I. The family unit is probably the most important source of support together with the specialist team. The team should not only be accessible and compassionate but should be prepared to offer referral to other sources of support, both financial and spiritual.

7 Treatment of leukemias, lymphomas and myelomas: current practice

Treatment is usually given soon after diagnosis for patients with all kinds of acute leukemias, chronic myeloid leukemia (CML), high-grade lymphomas and myelomas and some patients with chronic lymphocytic leukemia (CLL) and low-grade lymphoma. In most patients with CLL and low-grade lymphoma, treatment is usually only required in the more advanced stages because there is no evidence that treatment early in the disease is beneficial. This is in keeping with the over twenty centuries old teachings of Hippocrates, who admonished doctors that, above all, they should do no harm to the patient.

Until just under two decades ago, the mainstay of all hematological cancer treatment was cytotoxic chemotherapy, radiotherapy (also known as radiation therapy) and immunotherapy. The use of monoclonal antibodies reactive with discrete subsets of normal and cancerous (malignant) hemopoietic cells has increased greatly in the last decade and in 1998 the first successful molecularly targeted therapy entered the clinic. The place of stem cell transplantation (also known as bone marrow and blood transplantation) in the management of hematological cancers is discussed in Chapter 9. Most cytotoxic chemotherapy drugs work by disrupting the ability of cancer cells to grow and multiply. They can be administered by several routes. When given by mouth, the drugs are rapidly absorbed into the bloodstream from the gut and carried throughout the body to reach the cancer cells. Drugs that cannot be given by mouth, either because they are destroyed in the stomach and gut or because they are not well absorbed, are injected into subcutaneous fat or muscles or infused directly into a vein; that way they reach cancer cells rapidly and can begin to work without delay.

All cytotoxic chemotherapy drugs have their own specific modes of action; some kill cancer cells only when they are multiplying, while others kill all cancer cells. They can be used singly or in groups that work together, referred to as combination chemotherapy. Most treatment plans for hematological cancers include combination chemotherapy and, occasionally, radiation therapy, immunotherapy and the newer treatments, monoclonal antibodies. The molecularly targeted therapies have revolutionized the way we treat cancers in general since they specifically target the underlying molecular defects or abnormalities which play a principal role in the development of that particular cancer, in contrast to the non-specific way in which most other anti-cancer treatments work.

The quantity of each drug used in a combination is calculated for each patient according to his or her height and weight. The amount of a particular drug that can be used also depends on a person's genotype (inherited genes), which determines how an individual reacts. Currently this field, known as pharmacogenomics, is still in its infancy but the potential is enormous. A person's genotype needs to be established only once for any given gene, because except for very rare spontaneous mutations, it does not change. As we develop our molecular tools further, we can anticipate pharmacogenomics to play an increasing role in the management of our patients with all kinds of ailments.

Currently many efforts are being directed to predict individual patient's response to specific drugs based on the growing number of reports confirming the use of DNA microarray to identify and validate specific genomic signatures specific to certain cancers (Figure 7.1). For example in April 2004, Izidore Lossos and colleagues from Stanford, California validated a six-gene signature, independent of the other established prognostic tool for lymphomas, the IPI score (see Chapter 5), that predicts the response to standard chemotherapy (Figure 7.2).

Cytotoxic chemotherapy drugs also do not discriminate accurately between normal and cancer cells, so all cells can be affected to some degree and considerable damage can occur to normal tissue in which cell division is rapid. Cells that are particularly susceptible are those in the lining of the mouth and gut, the skin and the bone marrow. Most of these side-effects are unpleasant but usually reversible and generally not serious. However, very rarely serious complications do happen, so it is sensible for all patients who require intensive combination therapy to be treated where expert medical help and a first-rate supportive care facility are available. The treatment tends to involve a multidisciplinary approach and in general tends to be long and, though largely outpatient based, requires frequent hospital admissions. Moreover, regular medical supervision will be required, quite possibly for life. The outlook is influenced mainly by age, presence or absence of co-existing medical conditions, and factors related to the biology of the disease. The goal of such a treatment plan is to reduce and eradicate the cancer cells while preserving normal cells.

For all intravenously administered treatment, it is crucial to have good vascular access. For patients with acute leukemias, the treatment tends to be intensive and an indwelling central venous catheter is desired. Catheters, such as the Hickman or Hohn catheters, are usually inserted by a specialist nurse, surgeon or a radiologist, using a local or a general anesthetic (Figure 7.3). These catheters are used for taking blood samples and for giving intravenous fluids, chemotherapy, antibiotics, nutritional support and blood products. The tip of the catheter is usually positioned at the entrance to the right atrium (the upper right-sided chamber of the heart, through which all

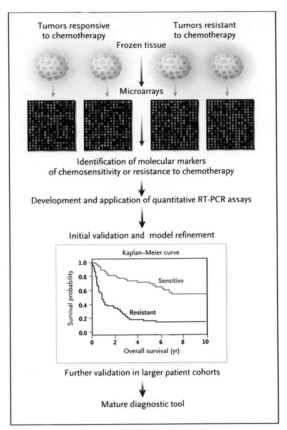

Figure 7.1   Development of DNA microarray-based diagnostic tests for cancer (reproduced with permission, from Ramaswamy S 2004, *N Engl J Med* 350: 1814–16).

the blood returns). In order to offer maximum use, most catheters comprise either double or triple tubes, each for injection of different materials. These catheters can remain in place for periods of 6 to 9 months, and sometimes even longer, without any complications. They do, however, require careful maintenance, particularly when home care is required. Patients are taught not only to change dressings but also flushing methods, in order to keep the tubes open (patent). Activities such as bathing, swimming, sexual intercourse, etc. can be enjoyed without any risk of damaging the catheter.

Sometimes specialists select a catheter which is connected to a small implantable port (such as Port-A-Cath; Figure 7.3(a)). This is a device implanted underneath the skin (subcutaneously) and is particularly suitable for patients receiving less-intensive treatment, and, perhaps, not as many blood products, such as patients with certain subtypes of high-grade lymphomas and myelomas. Most implantable ports have a single tube or lumen,

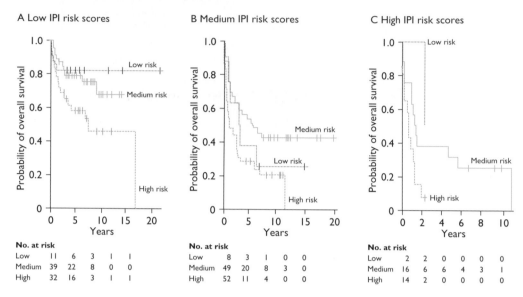

Figure 7.2   Predication of survival in diffuse large B-cell lymphoma: relationship between DNA microarray signatures and the IPI scores (reproduced with permission, from Lossos *et al.* (2004) *N Engl J Med* 350: 1828–37).

but double lumen ports are also available. The main advantage of these devices compared with the external catheters, such as Hickman, are the ease of maintenance and cosmetic appearance. They are also appealing to parents with young children, who can often pull the external catheters out with great ease, if allowed to!

Patients with hematological cancers might seek medical help because of an emergency such as life-threatening bleeding, a serious infection, a stroke (cerebrovascular accident – CVA) as a result of a very high blood count or a paralysis because of a mass or swelling compromising the spinal cord. In this

(a)   (b)

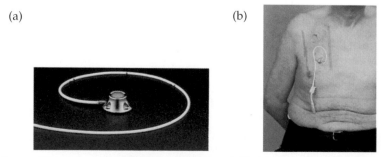

Figure 7.3   (a) A PORT-A-CATH® and (b) A Hickman catheter inserted in a patient with myeloma.

case these problems often have to be dealt with before specific anti-cancer therapy can be given. Infections are a particular problem with all hematological cancers and in particular patients with acute leukemias, CLL and myelomas. Over 50% of patients with these diseases tend to present with symptoms of an infection. Most patients, in particular those with acute leukemias, will require blood transfusions, usually of red blood cells and platelets. Today, all blood products, after being carefully screened for infectious diseases such as hepatitis A, B and C, HIV and HTLV-1, are filtered in order to reduce the chances of being contaminated by white blood cells which can result in allergic and febrile transfusion reactions. Most, if not all, blood products will also be irradiated in order to destroy any lymphocytes of donor origin which might be present in transfused blood and could mount a harmful reaction against the recipient, called graft-versus-host (GvH) reaction. This will be discussed in Chapter 9 which deals with stem cell transplantation. Irradiation of blood products before they are administered to the patient has been proven to be quite safe.

Leukemias

Acute myeloid leukemia

For patients with AML there are two sequential objectives of current standard treatment. The first is to induce a complete remission and the second is to prevent relapse. A complete remission is often defined as a state of a complete recovery of peripheral blood counts and the presence of less than 3% blasts in the bone marrow. The use of immunologic, cytogenetic and molecular genetic markers should improve on these definitions of complete remission in the future. The conventional treatment plan for all patients with AML consists of remission induction followed by post-remission therapy (consolidation therapy). It is now appropriate not to consider all patients with AML as a single entity for therapy, but rather to tailor this according to the individual risk category defined by cytogenetic and molecular criteria. This approach is epitomized by the subtype, acute promyelocytic leukemia (APL; M3), which is now the most curable subtype.

Remission induction

Substantial improvements have been made during the past two decades with regard to the proportion of patients under the age of 60 years who are able to achieve complete remission. These improvements appear to be largely due to better supportive care, which has enabled the safer delivery of more intensive remission induction, particularly with high doses of cytarabine. A variety of induction regimens followed by consolidation treatment with or without prolonged maintenance has been extensively investigated and the results suggest that about 70% achieve a complete remission and, with post-remission therapy, 25–30% will remain in complete remission at 5 years. For patients who receive less-intensive post-remission therapy, only 10–15% will remain in complete remission at 5 years. One of the major unresolved goals, therefore, is to improve on the proportion of patients who can remain in long-term continuous remission, and perhaps cure.

The most common remission induction consists of two courses of an anthracyline, usually daunorubicin, for 3 days and a continuous infusion of cytarabine for 7 days. Several randomized trials of alternatives to daunorubicin have suggested that both idarubicin and mitozantrone (mitoxantrone; Novantrone) are more effective, although both result in longer periods of pancytopenia. There is, however, some debate with regard to the equivalent doses and further studies are in progress. Daunorubicin is an anthracycline that acts directly by inhibiting cell growth by blocking the action of the enzyme topoisomerase II. Drugs which inhibit this powerful enzyme prevent repair of broken strands, resulting in cell death. It gives the urine a harmless reddish color which may persist for 24 to 48 hours, following the administration of the drug. It has several common side-effects including nausea, vomiting and bone marrow depression, which are discussed in Chapter 10. On rare occasions, it can also damage the heart muscle, particularly if given in a large amount. Specialists are therefore careful not to give too large a dose, or they may use an experimental drug concomitantly, such as Cardioxane, which functions as a cardioprotectant. Other efforts to minimize this effect have resulted in the recent introduction of a liposomal formulation of daunorubicin, Doxil, in the clinics.

Drugs such as idarubicin and epirubicin are the newer generation of anthra-cyclines. These agents appear less harmful to the heart and idarubicin also appears to be more potent in killing leukemia cells. Another related drug, mitozantrone, may also have fewer side-effects than daunorubicin. It belongs to another family (anthraquinones) but resembles anthracyclines in chemical structure and function. It has proven quite useful in the treatment of leukemias and may also have a role in lymphomas. All of these drugs can also produce substantial hair loss which may begin a week after the first injection. The amount of hair lost varies from individual to individual and is usually restricted to the scalp, although pubic, armpit and facial hair may also be affected. In almost all cases, the hair grows back completely and this is discussed in Chapter 10.

There has been considerable debate among specialists with regard to the merits of adding a third drug, often etoposide, to the remission induction treatment. Its merits are not well documented, except in patients with the subtypes M4 and M5. It is possible that by adding a fourth drug, usually 6-thioguanine, the success rate might improve, although this also has not been proven. 6-Thioguanine, which is relatively free of side-effects, works by stopping cells from making DNA.

Cytarabine (cystosine arabinoside; Ara-C) works by preventing leukemia cells from making DNA. It has very few harmful effects when used at conventional doses, and most patients tolerate it very well. Some patients may experience an 'Ara-C syndrome' where they develop fever, muscle aches, joint and bone pains, chest pain and eye toxicity. Very rarely, cytaribine causes a 'pulmonary syndrome' whereby patients develop diffuse lung abnormalities, sometimes resulting in respiratory failure. The rare side-effects might occur more frequently when higher doses (over $2g/m^2$) are used and with increasing age of the patients. At higher doses it sometimes also produces seizures (fits) and tremors, but these are fully reversible.

Most patients receive 1 or 2 cycles of induction therapy and then receive post-remission therapy which often includes a cycle of anthracycline (for 2 days) and cytarabine for 5 days followed by 2 to 4 cycles of high-dose cytarabine. In an attempt to improve the overall survival, several trials have incorporated higher doses of cytarabine (3 g/m^2, compared with the conventional 100 to 200 mg/m^2) in the induction phase. The overall survival in such studies, such as the UK-MRC-AML-12 trial, which recruited 2400 patients, has improved to 49%, but the toxicity from the high-dose cytarabine is considerable. In order to add further anti-leukemia treatment while limiting toxicity, some of the current trials (for example the UK-MRC-AML-15 trial) use antibody-directed chemotherapy. Gemtuzumab ozogamicin (Mylotarg; GO) is a novel agent which comprises a humanized monoclonal antibody directed against the CD33 molecule expressed on the surface of leukemia blasts in over 90% of patients with AML linked to calicheamycin, a very potent cell toxin. Gemtuzumab has been reported to have a few potentially serious side-effects and patients need to be observed carefully as we gain further experience. In the initial studies, there was a high incidence of infusion-related symptoms, such as skin rashes, cough, breathing difficulties, fevers and low blood pressure; all of these effects were fully reversible. It is also associated with liver toxicity, resembling veno-occlusive disease, which is usually seen after a stem cell transplant (see Chapter 9).

For patients with APL (AML-M3), remission induction consists of the drug all-*trans* retinoic acid (ATRA; tretinoin) plus an anthracycline-based regimen. ATRA works at the level of the mutated gene on chromosome 15. It probably binds to the abnormal protein produced by the mutated gene, altering the function of the protein. There is some uncertainty as to how best to combine ATRA with chemotherapy. Current evidence appears compelling that an anthracycline (daunorubicin or idarubicin) should be included in induction, since the APL cells appear to be fairly sensitive to anthracyclines; in contrast, cytarabine can probably be omitted. A recent study has shown that patients with APL fare just as well without cytarabine as part of their induction or consolidation treatment. The European APL group is addressing this issue further with patients being randomized to receive further ATRA plus daunorubicin or ATRA plus daunorubicin and cytarabine. There have been no randomized trials addressing the choice of anthracyclines so far, though there is agreement about the dose. It is reasonable to commence induction with ATRA alone for 2 to 4 days, provided the white blood count is not high, as it is remarkably effective in controlling the characteristic coagulopathy (a paradoxical bleeding–clotting disorder), which can often be life threatening and then commence anthracycline treatment. Earlier studies did suggest complete remission rates of about 80 to 90% with ATRA alone, but the remissions were shorter than those produced by ATRA followed by chemotherapy or chemotherapy alone. Despite the qualified success of ATRA, the mortality associated with the induction therapy remains at around 10% and an acquired retinoid resistance contributes to relapse in about 20 to 30% of patients. Current studies should show how best to integrate this novel molecular targeting and conventional chemotherapy.

ATRA does have a number of unique side-effects. Most patients experience a dry skin and their white blood count rises rapidly for a while, occasionally approaching 100×10^9/liter or more. This is in contrast to conventional induction therapy in which the counts decrease rapidly and in which bone marrow hypoplasia appears essential for a remission. This unique feature implies that remission has occurred as a consequence of the leukemia cells becoming differentiated and mature. ATRA does have a serious side-effect whereby a few patients may develop fever, low blood pressure, very high white cell counts and abnormal lungs (infiltrates). The lining of the heart (the pericardium) can become water-logged (pericardial effusion) in rare instances. These effects are known as the capillary leak syndrome (referred to as the ATRA syndrome) and are usually completely reversible.

Consolidation (post-remission) therapy

All patients under the age of 60 years who achieve a complete remission following induction therapy require further treatment in order to improve their chances of remaining in continuous complete remission. Currently there are three well-defined and intensively investigated options of either receiving an allogeneic stem cell transplant from an HLA-matched donor (sibling or unrelated) or an autologous stem cell transplant, or further intensive chemotherapy. We will discuss the transplant aspects in Chapter 9. Several large studies have shown that patients treated with several (2 to 4) cycles of high-dose cytarabine may fare just as well as those subjected to a transplant, autologous or allogeneic, during first remission of AML. A further recent study has demonstrated evidence of a dose–response effect of cytarabine in patients with AML, including those in the poor-risk group.

These studies have introduced an element of uncertainty as to how best to treat patients under the age of 60 years who are in first complete remission. It would appear reasonable not to offer an allogeneic stem cell transplant as first-line post-remission treatment to all patients, but rather in accordance to their risk category and, preferably, in the context of clinical trials. Current comparative trials are assessing the potential improvements in autologous stem cell transplant by better engraftment with the use of peripheral blood stem cells and it should be possible to better identify patients who can benefit from salvage transplantation.

For patients who relapse with AML, the treatment options are few. For patients in the good-risk group who relapse following a remission of at least 12 months, the survival rate following subsequent chemotherapy treatment is about 20%. For these reasons every effort is directed to prevent relapse. For children and adults younger than 40 years of age, it is reasonable to proceed with a stem cell transplant, either an autograft or an allograft using an HLA-matched sibling donor. It is uncertain as to whether these patients should first receive induction therapy or proceed directly with transplantation. An earlier study from the Seattle group assessed these aspects and showed an equivalent survival with either option. Current European Blood and Marrow Transplant (EBMT) registry data suggest a survival rate of about 30% for patients with AML in first relapse or second complete remission treated by an autologous or allogeneic stem cell transplant, using an HLA-identical sibling donor.

For patients with APL who enter complete remission, anthracycline-consolidation therapy is required, though there is some uncertainty with regards to the number of cycles needed. Studies have also suggested that all patients should receive maintenance therapy with ATRA, with or without low-dose chemotherapy. There is some concern with regard to the possible increased neurotoxicity associated with ATRA maintenance therapy, particularly in children. Therapy-related myelodysplastic syndrome (MDS) and secondary AML are also being increasingly recognized in patients with APL and better risk stratification and monitoring of residual disease by polymerase chain reaction should facilitate better individualization of therapies. Arsenic trioxide (Trisenox) is now considered effective treatment for those patients who relapse or are refractory to ATRA-based therapy. The role of arsenic trioxide during the induction phase is also being investigated, based on a synergism with ATRA.

Allogeneic stem cell transplant (SCT) has no role in the management of APL in first remission since the results from current induction treatments are excellent. Allogeneic SCT may be useful for patients who relapse following an arsenic trioxide-induced second complete remission (Chapter 9).

Treatment of patients older than 60 years of age with AML

This age group accounts for about 75% of patients with newly diagnosed AML, the majority of whom are in the poor-risk group. Furthermore older patients are less able to tolerate the rigors associated with the intensive induction regimens, let alone transplantation. Older patients are also much more likely to have an intrinsic resistance to chemotherapy making them less likely to respond as well as the younger patients. The incidence of significant co-morbid medical conditions is also high in this cohort. A nihilistic approach unfortunately results in a poor quality of life and very poor survival; therefore, every effort should be made to individualize therapy. Patients who are younger than 80 years of age, have no significant medical history and have a good performance status have an approximately 50% chance of achieving complete remission with conventional induction treatment and an event-free survival of about 20% at 2 years. A minority may benefit from low-dose maintenance therapy, in particular from the quality of life perspective. Many efforts are being devoted to improve the supportive care of these patients and to use hemopoietic growth factors, in particular granulocyte colony-stimulating factor (G-CSF), as an adjunct to induction therapy.

Other investigational therapies in AML

Considerable advances have been made in the molecular understanding of AML and some of this progress has resulted in being able to target the leukemia cells with molecular and immunologic strategies. The first successful example of this has been the use of ATRA in the treatment of APL. It is likely that novel agents targeting the P-glycoprotein and the multidrug resistance (MDR-1) gene will enter clinics in the near future. The impressive results obtained with the tyrosine kinase inhibitor, imatinib, for the treatment of patients with CML in myeloid blast crisis suggest that, with further molecular understanding, other novel therapies should emerge. Other potentially useful tyrosine kinase inhibitors in clinical studies include the FLT-3 and KIT inhibitors, such as the drug SU11248 which is directed against the high levels of these receptors found in AML. A related drug which inhibits the farnesyltransferase enzyme and thereby targets of the oncogene RAS, called tipifarnib (Zarnestra; R11577), has also recently entered clinical studies, with encouraging preliminary results.

Acute lymphoblastic leukemia

The conventional approach for all patients with acute lymphoblastic leukemia (ALL), except the mature B-cell subtype (FAB L3) and infants with ALL, is a treatment plan directed first at the destruction of all leukemia cells in the bone marrow and lymphoid system, and, second at destroying any leukemia cells that are left in 'sanctuary sites'. These are parts of the body, including the testes, ovaries, brain and spinal cord, where leukemia cells are found but where it is difficult to achieve high concentrations of antileukemic drugs. ALL cells, in contrast to AML cells, can reside in sanctuaries, in a resting state (G_0 phase; see Chapter 1) for prolonged periods before they begin proliferating again and cause a clinical relapse; rarely AML cells, in particular the monocytic variety, can behave in this manner. The treatment plan is usually divided into three phases: remission induction, consolidation and maintenance. All patients with ALL who achieve complete remission should receive some form of central nervous system (CNS) prophylaxis. The mature B-cell ALL and infant ALL appear to be best treated with short-term regimens of intensive therapy and will be addressed separately.

Remission induction

The principal aim is to achieve complete remission with restoration of normal hemopoiesis. Better supportive care has made it safer for patients with standard and poor-risk ALL to receive more intensive induction regimens with four or more drugs and current results suggest that over 95% of children and 75–90% of adults are able to achieve a complete remission and, with consolidation and maintenance therapy, about 80% of children and 30% of adults will remain in complete remission at 5 years.

Induction therapy typically includes prednisolone or dexamethasone, vincristine, L-asparaginase, daunorubicin or idarubicin, and sometimes cyclophosphamide. Once complete remission is achieved, several extra courses of the same drugs are given to minimize the likelihood of recurrence. This is referred to as consolidation (or post-remission) therapy.

Prednisolone belongs to the same family that includes anabolic steroids, which are often used illicitly by some athletes to boost their athletic performance (as was rather sadly reported among a few of the Athens Olympiad August 2004 athletes!). Prednisolone is given by mouth and can cause stomach upsets, particularly from superficial ulcers, and high blood pressure due to water retention. Rarely it can cause psychiatric difficulties, especially depression and other alterations of mood and thinking. In addition it can cause muscle cramps, blurred vision and difficulty in sleeping. In individuals who have diabetes, it often aggravates it by raising the blood sugar levels. However, its beneficial action is rapid and it has proven to be of exceptional value in acutely ill patients. It can also increase the appetite. The side-effects usually disappear when the drug is discontinued. Dexamethasone is a related drug which might confer a greater effect on cancer cells than prednisolone. It also has the advantage of penetrating the CNS more effectively.

Vincristine is a potent cytotoxic drug extracted from the periwinkle plant *Catharanthus (vinca) rosea*. It works directly on the cancer cells by binding to the protein tubulin and preventing cell division. Tubulin forms fibers that help cell division to progress in an orderly fashion. Since all leukemia cells do not divide at the same time, vincristine is given weekly in the hope that eventually all the cells will be affected. Vincristine can cause constipation and stomach cramps and rarely paresthesias (neuropathy). Given in excess, it can lead to temporary paralysis of the bowel or of certain nerves, resulting in muscle weakness which may result in foot-drop, wrist-drop and facial paralysis. Most of these effects are completely reversible and are rarely seen in current treatment schedules.

L-Asparaginase works by depriving cancer cells of an essential food stuff, an amino acid called asparagine. Several forms of asparaginase, each with a different pharmokinetic profile, are currently available. In a single randomized study patients treated with asparaginase derived from *Escherichia coli* fared better than that derived from *Erwinia carotovora*. They can all produce allergic reactions and, less frequently, inflammation of the liver and pancreas. The allergic reactions are sometimes quite serious and can cause difficulty in breathing, or a puffy face and rashes. Other side-effects include tiredness, loss of appetite, stomach cramps and an increase in the amount of sugar in the blood. The latter effect can simulate diabetes and cause frequent urination and increased thirst. Rarely it can result in thrombosis by altering the synthesis of many of the proteins involved in the body's coagulation process.

All patients with ALL who achieve complete remission should receive some form of proven CNS prophylaxis. The standard approach is to administer cranial irradiation totalling 1800 cGy in conjunction with intrathecal methotrexate. Recent experiences suggest that the dose of cranial irradiation can safely be reduced to 1200 cGy, even in patients at high risk. This lower dose of irradiation could be valuable in reducing the risk of late cerebral toxicity. Intrathecal methotrexate without irradiation has resulted in comparatively high rates of CNS relapse and it is possible that methotrexate in combination with cytarabine and dexamethasone (triple intrathecal therapy) might be better. Moreover since most induction regimens nowadays include drugs which are able to cross the blood–brain barrier, it is likely that the need for additional irradiation may have diminished. Recently, however, the results of the Boston-ALL consortium protocol at a median follow-up of 9.2 years suggested that eliminating cranial irradiation without a concomitant increased intensity of systemic or intrathecal therapy results in a marked increase in CNS relapse in standard-risk male children, but interestingly not female children.

Parenthetically it should be emphasized that as attempts have been made to increase the intensity of the remission induction, complex regimens using multiple drugs have entered the clinics at frequent intervals without being tested stringently in randomized trials. This has made it difficult to assess with any precision the results of the more intensive treatments, nor is it possible to draw firm opinions on the contributions of each individual drug. These points notwithstanding, most current treatment protocols are well received by the specialists in view of the improving outcomes of the patients.

For patients with mature B-cell ALL the prognosis is poor for both children and adults and, as recently as a decade ago, the probability of achieving a complete remission was about 35%. Newer treatment strategies based on experiences from the treatment of children and young adults with Burkitt's lymphoma resulted in the inclusion of fractionated high-dose cyclophosphamide, high-dose methotrexate, and cytarabine (standard dose). These modifications led to the complete remission rates improving to 75% and the event-free survival to around 50%. These improvements have been credited to the high-dose components of the protocols although it is difficult to assess which of the high-dose combinations are more important and the optimal doses remain debatable. Further refinements have occurred since and the currently reported complete remission rate is 85%. Once a complete remission is achieved it appears desirable to proceed with an intensive consolidation for about 8 months. Neither autologous nor allogeneic SCT have been tested adequately but should be considered, in the context of a clinical trial, for patients who fail to achieve a complete remission with one or two induction treatments. Maintenance therapy appears to have no value in this disease. Since the high-dose drugs used are active in CNS disease, patients receive additional intrathecal methotrexate without cranial irradiation.

Methotrexate works by preventing cells from making new DNA by blocking the enzyme *dihydrofolate reductase*. It can be given by mouth in small doses since it is absorbed well and excreted rapidly by normally functioning kidneys. Higher doses are given intravenously. In patients with impaired kidney function, methotrexate can accumulate very rapidly and result in side-effects, such as severe gut ulcerations. It can also cause hair loss, skin eruptions and liver damage, and even lung damage can occur.

Cyclophosphamide is a very useful drug in the treatment of almost all hematological cancers. It is a 'prodrug' and therefore requires activation by liver enzymes before it can work. It works by binding to the cellular DNA and prevents it from uncoiling and therefore replicating.

Patients with Ph-positive ALL tend to have a very poor prognosis. Recent results of incorporating imatinib in the treatment plan, after complete remission has been achieved, appear quite encouraging. For the moment, however, most specialists favor the approach of subjecting all such patients to an allogeneic stem cell transplant (SCT) once they have achieved a complete remission with chemotherapy. Post-transplant studies are assessing the benefit of maintenance imatinib.

Post-remission therapy

Once remission is achieved and normal hemopoiesis restored, therapy is continued in accordance with one or other established schedule. Most schedules incorporate the use of daily 6-mercaptopurine and weekly oral methotrexate concomitantly with a once-monthly dose of alternating daunorubicin, vincristine and cyclophosphamide or a similar alternative schedule. 6-Mercaptopurine works by interfering with the synthesis of the building blocks of DNA. It is relatively free of major side-effects; toxicity, when seen, is largely due to the suppression of the bone marrow. It can also cause abnormal liver function, although this is rare. Some specialists prefer to use a more intensive regimen, in particular for the poor risk category and there is no definite agreement on the optimal schedule or the optimal duration, although the usefulness of this phase of the treatment is established, even in patients with low-risk disease. Its value, however, is less certain in adults with poor-risk disease and there is a trend to offer this cohort of patients a more intensive multidrug therapy.

Following the completion of consolidation therapy, the optimal duration of which (as discussed above) remains uncertain, most patients in continuous complete remission, with the exception of those with mature B-cell phenotype, receive prolonged treatment for a further few years. The validity of such an approach remains unclear but most specialists are of the opinion that long-term multidrug exposure may aid in destroying the residual leukemia cells or assist in apoptosis. A recent meta-analysis of trials assessing maintenance therapy concluded that it was probably valuable, but not beyond a period of 3 years.

Treatment of relapsed ALL

Despite the significant improvement in the therapy of ALL, in particular in children, about 25% of children and 60% of adults experience a relapse. A second remission can be achieved in most of these patients, but in many cases it is not sustained. Factors which are associated with a poor outcome after a relapse include a shorter length of first remission, bone marrow as the initial site of relapse, older age, T-cell ALL and male sex. A UK-MRC-ALL study showed that patients who had a bone marrow relapse during the first 24 months following their initial diagnosis fare the worst. This study showed that patients with an isolated extramedullary relapse do have a better prognosis, even though many will have molecular evidence of bone marrow relapse. This study also showed that only 3% of patients with a bone marrow relapse are alive in second remission at 5 years irrespective of the type of their second treatment. There is considerable uncertainty with regards to the appropriate further treatment once a second remission is established. There have been no prospective randomized trials of second post-remission chemotherapy versus stem cell transplant so the evidence available is largely based on comparison with historical controls.

Notwithstanding the good results of intensive chemotherapy in children with good- and standard-risk ALL, the treatment of the remaining children and most adults remains relatively difficult. Substantial efforts are being directed to improve this scenario, both in terms of understanding the molecular pathogenesis better and new therapeutic agents in addition to the potential role of stem cell transplantation (Chapter 9). One particular drug, arabinosylguanine (Compound 506U) has shown encouraging activity in T-cell ALL.

Chronic myeloid leukemia

The management of CML epitomizes the art of shared decision making whereby the specialist gives the patient factual information about available treatment options, the probability of benefits and the morbidity, and the degree of scientific evidence. This strategy has gained support as both transplant and non-transplant therapy for CML in chronic phase have improved over the past decade and the real objectives in the management need to be addressed. It is prudent to discuss the relative merits of imatinib, IFN-α and allogeneic stem cell transplant with the patient at the time of diagnosis. There is good evidence that some patients can be cured by allogeneic SCT and various methods have been designed to develop a risk score that can predict within broad limits the probability of survival and transplant-related mortality for individual patients. In contrast the management of patients with the advanced phases of CML tends to be similar to that of the poor risk acute leukemias.

Imatinib mesylate

Imatinib mesylate was thought to work uniquely by occupying the 'kinase' pocket of the BCR-ABL oncoprotein and blocking access to an important molecule (ATP), thereby preventing 'phosphorylation' of any substrate and so inhibiting the activity of the oncoprotein; it is now thought to act in part by binding to an adjacent domain in a manner that holds the Abl component of the BCR-ABL oncoprotein in an inactive configuration (Figure 7.4). Imatinib entered clinical trials in 1998 and its efficacy in conferring

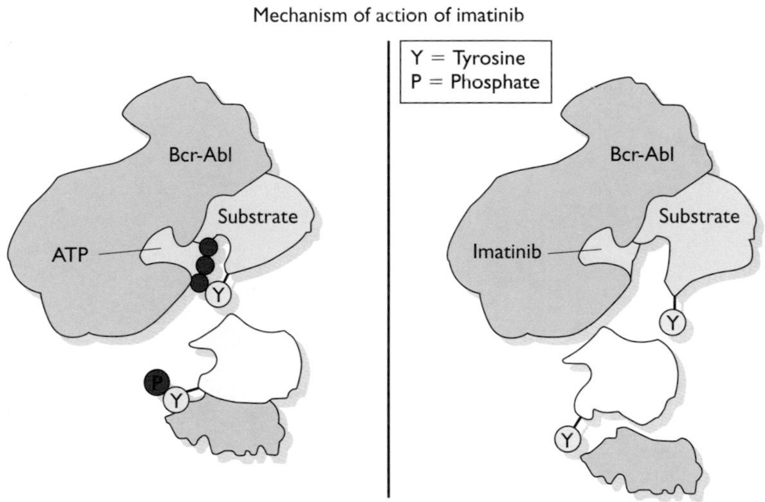

Mechanism of action of imatinib

Y = Tyrosine
P = Phosphate

Figure 7.4   A schematic representation of how imatinib works [reproduced with permission from Mughal and Goldman (2004) Chronic myeloid leukemia: current status and controversies, *Oncology* 18: 837–53].

127

hematological (return of blood counts to normal) and cytogenetic (loss of the Ph chromosome) responses was established fairly quickly. By summer 2001, the drug was granted regulatory approval, initially by the FDA and soon afterwards the European agencies. Current results confirm the initial impressive results of imatinib. Notably, over 95% of patients with CML in chronic phase achieve a complete hematological response, and 74% of these patients achieve a major cytogenetic response, but thus for only a few patients have achieved convincing molecular remissions (Figure 7.5). It is, however, not possible to conclude that imatinib as a single agent cures substantial numbers of patients, but it may well offer the prospect of 'operational cure' to a significant proportion.

Although imatinib appears to be quite safe, caution must be exercised in the light of several recent reports. A Swiss group has reported a fatal development of cerebral edema soon after the initiation of imatinib therapy. A French group reported an interesting observation of hair repigmentation. In most cases the side-effects are relatively minor and infrequent. Some patients developed cytopenias (low blood counts) and abnormal liver tests; rashes, generalized bone pains and fluid retention are seen in about 5% of the patients. A recent report suggested a possible effect on male fertility by causing a reduction in the sperm count. More studies are needed to confirm this.

Imatinib has also proven to be active in patients with the more advanced phases of CML, though in most cases the benefits have been relatively short-lived. Studies are now assessing the candidacy of imatinib as combination therapy,

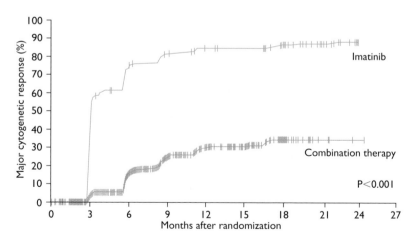

Figure 7.5   Results of a study comparing imatinib with interferon alfa and cytarabine as initial therapy for patients with chronic myeloid leukemia [reproduced with permission from O'Brien *et al.* (2003) Interferon and low-dose cytarabine in newly diagnosed chronic myeloid leukemia, *N Engl J Med* 348: 994–1004].

combined with cytarabine and other cytotoxic drugs. Some laboratory studies suggest some antagonism between imatinib and IFN-α and hydroxyurea.

A major concern regarding imatinib therapy is the development of resistance. The most common cause of resistance appears to be acquired mutations in the *BCR-ABL* gene (in the kinase region). The risk of mutation development is particularly high in patients who are in the advanced phases of the disease as well as those with a long duration of chronic phase disease prior to imatinib therapy. Other mechanisms, mentioned briefly in Chapter 7, include the CML cells evading imatinib's inhibitory effects by other diverse mechanisms, including overexpression of the oncoprotein as a possible consequence of *BCR-ABL* gene amplification, P-glycoprotein overexpression resulting in reduction in the uptake of imatinib, and possibly excessive degradation of the oncoprotein. There is a great deal of research activity in progress assessing different strategies to overcome resistance to imatinib. One such strategy, which was very recently noted to be promising, is combining drugs called flavopiridol and bortezomib (Velcade) to treat patients with CML resistant to imatinib. This combination appears to work by inducing apoptosis. We discuss other newer therapeutic approaches below.

Interferon-alfa

IFN-α (Intron-A, Roferon-A) treatment was until recently the mainstay of treatment for CML. It is part of the interferon family and is a protein (synthesized by recombinant DNA technology) with antiviral, antiproliferative and other properties which can affect the immune system in various ways. IFN-α was available in the late 1970s and entered clinical trials in the 1980s. In the mid-1990s it was established as the non-transplant treatment of choice for patients with CML in the chronic phase, following several clinical trials comparing IFN-α with hydroxyurea and busulfan, which were the standard treatment from the 1950s to the early 1980s. It induced hematological responses in about 80% of patients and major cytogenetic responses in about 35% and an overall survival advantage of 1 to 2 years compared with hydroxyurea. There were very few documented molecular remissions. It was noteworthy, however, that many of the patients responding were able to continue their normal day to day activity and a small proportion did not require any specific therapy for their CML and could be classified as 'operationally cured'; a 'formal' cure was eluded since they all had disease at a molecular level. In molecular biology parlance an 'operational cure' would imply a low number of leukemia cells which persist but appear unable to re-establish clinical disease.

There are several important issues still unresolved with regard to IFN-α. The optimal dose remains a matter of some controversy, with the average weekly doses ranging from 9 MU to 35 MU or more. Moreover the duration of IFN-α treatment remains undefined. Side-effects are mild in general but quite common. Most patients suffer from flu-like symptoms, lethargy and weight loss; less common side-effects include immune-mediated complications, such as thrombocytopenia and hypothyroidism. In an attempt to reduce this toxicity, specialists began using a long-acting form of the drug, pegylated IFN-α. The notion of adding cytarabine to IFN-α appeared attractive on the basis of several studies completed in the early 2000s and, by 2001, many specialists felt that initial treatment for newly diagnosed patients with CML in chronic phase should be with IFN-α and cytarabine. This view has now been eclipsed by the introduction of imatinib.

Hydroxyurea

Hydroxyurea (hydroxycarbamide; Hydrea; Mylocel) works by inhibiting the enzyme *RNA reductase* and interfering with protein synthesis. It became the standard treatment for CML in the early 1980s, when the toxicity of busulfan (Myleran), in particular the pulmonary fibrosis and irreversible gonodal failure, was recognized. The drug is given by mouth and works fairly rapidly, usually restoring the spleen size and blood counts to normal within 4 to 8 weeks. Treatment may be maintained for many years. Side-effects are rare but include mouth ulcers, rashes, leg ulcers and various gastrointestinal upsets. All the side-effects are completely reversible on stopping the drug. The drug remains valuable today for rapid reduction of the leukemia cell numbers in the newly diagnosed patient. It is also of considerable value in the management of elderly patients who might not be able to tolerate imatinib because of possible fluid retention and also those who simply cannot afford to receive imatinib or IFN-α.

Newer therapeutic approaches

The demonstration that imatinib durably blocks the kinase activity of the BCR-ABL oncoprotein has provided a major incentive for the development of a second generation of kinase inhibitors. One such agent, dasatinib (Bristol Myers Squibb Pharma), has a chemical structure rather different from that of imatinib and appears to inhibit the kinase activity of both the ABL and SRC gene products. Preliminary clinical experience suggests that it is active against leukemia cells from patients who have developed resistance to imatinib as a consequence of expanded clones with kinase domain mutations. Similarly, the new ABL inhibitor designated AMN107 (Novartis Pharma) is proving to be active in imatinib-resistant cell lines. It is likely that other analogous kinase inhibitors will become available before long. It would be logical to test such new agents in combinations with imatinib.

In February 2005, another small molecule, ON012380 (Onconova Therapeutics), was noted to be a potent inhibitor of BCR-ABL. This molecule works differently from imatinib and acts synergistically with imatinib in vitro. It entered clinical trials in August 2005.

The demonstration of a powerful graft-versus-leukemia (GvL) effect in CML following an allogeneic transplant (See chapter 9) has renewed interest in the possibility that some form of immunotherapeutic manipulation could be effective in CML. Some evidence suggests that patients vaccinated with oligopeptides corresponding to the junctional region of the BCR-ABL protein may generate immune responses that may be of clinical benefit. Other potential targets for vaccine therapy now under study include the Wilms tumor-1 protein and proteinase-3, both of which are overexpressed in CML cells.

Chronic lymphocytic leukemia

Some patients with CLL have an indolent disease and may not require any specific therapy since this would not prolong survival, though over 50% of all patients with early-stage CLL do eventually progress and require treatment. Most specialists offer treatment when patients present with more advanced disease. It may also be desirable to begin treatment when patients develop 'B' symptoms (weight loss, fevers, night sweats), there is progressive evidence of increasing tumor burden, such as increasing white cell count, enlarging lymph nodes and spleen enlargement. It is noteworthy that over 50% of patients with CLL experience recurrent infections, which are often exacerbated by some of the treatments used (see below).

Chlorambucil (Leukeran), either alone or with a steroid, usually prednisolone, has been the most frequently used first-line drug in the treatment of CLL for almost four decades. Cyclophosphamide (Cytoxan) orally is an equivalent drug. For patients presenting with more advanced disease, combination chemotherapy is often resorted to. The most common regimens are cyclophosphamide, vincristine and prednisolone; sometimes an anthracycline is also added. Although these latter regimens have resulted in higher responses, there are no major durable responses or survival advantages compared with chlorambucil. A recent meta-analysis on data collated by the UK-CLL-Trialists' Collaborative Group validates these observations and confirmed no survival advantages for immediate versus deferred chemotherapy in patients with early-stage CLL. There has, however, been some debate with regard to these conclusions, since few of the studied patients had been treated with fludarabine.

Fludarabine (Fludara) is a purine analog, which was found in 1990 to be a remarkably effective treatment for patients with CLL resistant to chorambucil. It works by inhibiting DNA synthesis and promoting apoptosis in CLL cells. Thereafter there was much enthusiasm with regard to using this drug as a first-line therapy and a number of clinical trials were embarked upon. In 1996 the results of the first randomized US trial comparing fludarabine with chlorambucil in patients with newly diagnosed CLL confirmed a higher incidence of both complete remissions and overall responses, but no evidence of prolongation of survival. A smaller French study of fludarabine versus combination chemotherapy (cyclophosphamide, daunorubicin and prednisolone) revealed a similar finding. These and other studies have led some specialists to use fludarabine as a first-line therapy while others prefer to use it as a second-line, pending the results of further ongoing studies.

Fludarabine is quite toxic to the bone marrow and the immune system in view of its profound depletion of T lymphocytes and associated increased risk of viral and fungal infections. It can be given by mouth or intravenously with equal efficacy and equivalent side-effect profile (currently only the intravenous form is available in the US). Specialists are also investigating the potential role of two other drugs, cladribine and pentostatin, in the treatment of CLL refractory to the above therapies. Both these drugs are chemically related to fludarabine and currently have an established role in the treatment of patients with hairy cell leukemia, which we discuss below. We discuss the potential role of stem cell transplant, in particular for the younger patients, in Chapter 9.

Other investigational therapies include the use of monoclonal antibodies, in particular alemtuzumab (Campath-1H) and rituximab (Rituxan; Mabthera). These agents work by binding to the cancer cells, following their intravenous administration, and recruit the host immune system against these antibody-bound cancer cells. Campath-1H is a humanized rat antibody against the antigen CD52 found on malignant B and T lymphocytes and other normal cells. It is the first antibody to be approved by the FDA for the treatment of patients with CLL refractory to chlorambucil and/or fludarabine, on the basis of a 33% response rate in a small study of 93 patients who had progressed after receiving chlorambucil or cyclophosphamide and failed to respond to fludarabine. Current studies are assessing the role of Campath-1H as first-line therapy compared with chlorambucil. Combination therapy of fludarabine, Campath-1H and rituximab is also being considered as a potential investigational second-line treatment based on small pilot studies. Campath-1H is also being investigated as a purging agent in patients being considered for autologous stem cell transplant (see Chapter 9). Rituximab is currently approved for treatment of low-grade lymphomas, but following a number of small studies was found to have some activity in patients with CLL. This was somewhat surprising since most patients have low levels of the surface antigen CD20 (on B cells), the principal target for rituximab. Significantly increased activity has been reported by some specialists who have combined this agent with fludarabine and cyclophosphamide. It is possible that rituximab works in CLL by some other mechanism. There has been some evidence that it 'down regulates' the BCL-2 gene which plays a role in CLL.

In the rare subtype, T-cell CLL, which represents less than 3% of all European and US patients with CLL, but is the dominant form of CLL in Asia, patients often present with low blood counts (pancytopenia) and prominent splenomegaly; the lack of lymphadenopathy is noteworthy. The general prognosis is similar to poor-risk CLL and most patients tend to be refractory to chlorambucil and fludarabine treatment.

Radiotherapy is occasionally used to relieve symptoms produced by bulky lymph nodes or an enormously enlarged spleen. In the past total-body irradiation was sometimes used but it is now not used because of the resulting bone marrow suppression.

Prolymphocytic leukemia (PLL)

Most patients with PLL have a clinical course similar to poor-risk CLL and do respond to an anthracycline-containing chemotherapy combination or fludarabine. A minority of patients have an indolent course.

Large granular lymphocytic (LGL) leukemia

The majority of patients with LGL leukemia do not require any specific treatment at presentation and various strategies have been offered on an *ad hoc* basis, including prednisolone, cyclophosphamide (low dose), IFN-α, splenectomy and intensive chemotherapy for the more aggressive forms. The prognostic factors associated with poor prognosis are fever, low CD56 expression and low granular lymphocyte counts.

Hairy cell leukemia

Most patients with hairy cell leukemia require treatment. In less than 10% of patients, who are elderly and have an impalpable spleen, the course is indolent and no treatment may be required. In the past splenectomy was the initial choice and almost all patients benefited for at least a few months, largely owing to fewer infections and lesser blood transfusion requirements. Unfortunately most develop progressive disease and require other therapies. In the late 1980s, interferon alfa (IFN-α) became the mainstay treatment with over 90% of all patients showing a substantial benefit. Most patients enjoy long periods of remission, but many relapse when therapy is discontinued. Moreover IFN-α is administered subcutaneously three times (or more) and associated with a number of mild, but frequent, side-effects.

The use of the purine analogs, cladribine (2-chlorodeoxyadenosine; 2-CdA) and pentostatin (2-deoxycoformycin; Nipent), over the past decade has dramatically improved the overall scenario for patients with hairy cell leukemia and introduced the possibility of a cure for these patients. Both these drugs result in almost 95% complete responses and the responses appear to be long lasting. There have been no comparative randomized trials comparing these two drugs, and it is acceptable to use either as a first-line therapy. Most specialists (and patients) prefer cladribine simply because it is administered in a single course as a continuous intravenous infusion over 5 to 7 days. Very few patients require a second cycle. It has few side-effects, other than bone marrow suppression resulting in neutropenia, which is maximal a week after the therapy. Pentostatin is administered as an intravenous infusion every 14 days until a maximum response is observed in the bone marrow and then two additional cycles are administered.

A subtle transformation sometime takes place in patients with hairy cell leukemia in the form of massive abdominal lymph nodes and resistance to cladrabine, pentostatin and IFN-α treatments. The prognosis is often serious.

Adult T-cell leukemia/lymphoma

Standard therapy of adult T-cell leukemia/lymphoma (ATLL) is similar to that employed in the management of poor-prognosis high-grade lymphoma, but the outcome is generally unsatisfactory. Allogeneic SCT could be contemplated if a suitable donor is available.

Myelodysplastic syndrome

At present an allogeneic stem cell transplant is the only form of treatment which has the potential to cure patients with myelodysplastic syndrome (MDS), but the optimal timing of the transplant is not known (we discuss this in Chapter 9). A recent analysis from the Center for International Bone Marrow Transplant Registry (CIBMTR) suggested an early transplant for patients with high-risk MDS and a delayed transplant, but prior to leukemia progression and probably at the time of the emergence of a new cytogenetic abnormality, for the cohort with low- and intermediate-risk disease. This strategy was shown to result in maximal life expectancy for all patients. Once MDS has transformed into acute leukemia, standard AML-type chemotherapy often gives unsatisfactory results and the prognosis tends to be poor. It is often best to treat patients with MDS in accordance to their prognostic score. It is of interest to note that when patients are stratified in this way, there are no major differences between the outcome of patients with MDS and AML with an equivalent cytogenetic abnormality; patients with MDS are, however, much more likely to have poor prognostic disease profiles. Patients with deletions in chromosome 7 and trisomy 8 appear to fare particularly badly. In contrast patients with 5q− syndrome can often be maintained on supportive red blood cell transfusions alone for long periods. Induction chemotherapy regimens containing some of the newer drugs, such as topotecan, have shown encouraging responses, as have several new investigational approaches. The new thalidomide analogue, Lenalidomide (Revlimid; CC-50/3) has shown encouraging durable responses in patients with the 5q-subtype of MDS and is expected to be approved by the FDA for this indication in November 2005.

For patients with MDS who are totally asymptomatic, there is often no urgency to commence therapy, unless they wish to be subjected to a stem cell transplant and have a suitable donor available or wish to participate in a clinical trial. Patients with mild asymptomatic anemia and low platelet counts without evidence of bleeding do not require transfusion. However once patients become symptomatic or at risk for significant bleeding, they should be offered transfusion support, which is often the mainstay treatment for these patients.

A wide range of non-transplant treatments have been investigated over the past three decades, but sadly with very few data available to suggest that treatment of these patients results in a survival improvement. However, (importantly) some treatments may modify the natural history of and improve the quality of life for patients with MDS. Cytotoxic chemotherapeutic drugs have generally not fared well in these patients. The principal reasons for this are the relatively older age of patients with MDS, the higher prevalence of drug resistance due to increased expression of the MDR-1 gene, and the rather limited reserves of healthy bone marrow for recovery. Low-dose chemotherapy, largely with differentiating agents, such as low-dose cytarabine, 5-aza-2'-deoxycytidine (azacytidine; Vidaza), retinoids (ATRA) and cholecalciferols, have been assessed extensively based on *in vitro* observations that the blasts (myeloblasts) in MDS might be induced to differentiate and that remission might be achieved without a marrow aplasia. The results for the most part have been disappointing, but it is of interest that azacytidine was approved by the Food and Drug Administration (FDA) in the US for treatment of MDS in July 2004, largely in response to a small phase III trial where hematological benefit was observed in about 60% of patients with MDS allocated azacytidine therapy. Some activity has been observed in patients receiving ATRA with EPO and further studies are ongoing. There is still adequate scientific enthusiasm to support further clinical trials of differentiating agents in this disease. Immunotherapy has met a slightly higher degree of success in patients with MDS. The antithymocyte globulins were the primary immunotherapeutic agents in use prior to the advent of a variety of monoclonal antibodies against proteins expressed disproportionally on the myeloblasts.

For patients with the subtype chronic myelomonocytic leukemia (CMML), treatment with hydroxyurea is fairly effective in controlling the peripheral monocytosis, but not in producing complete remissions. It has also been noted that patients with CMML who have a reciprocal translocation involving chromosome 5q33 might be responsive to imatinib. Imatinib might work here on the platelet-derived growth factor receptor (PDGFR) and further studies are in progress. Very recently it has been shown in studies that mouse models with CMML can achieve complete remissions with a drug called SU11657. Another potentially useful drug is AMG 706 (Amgen), which works by inhibiting a number of tyrosine kinases and is also an anti-angiogenesis agent.

Hemopoietic growth factors, both G-CSF and GM-CSF, have been investigated and found to be moderately useful in the correction of neutropenias, but most cytopenias returned to their pre-therapy levels once the growth factors were discontinued. Currently combinations of G-CSF or GM-CSF, erythropoietin, stem cell factor and in some cases, differentiating agents are being evaluated. Parenthetically, some concern was expressed recently following the observation of increasing blasts in a cohort of patients receiving G-CSF compared with a placebo, but further studies have confirmed that short-term (often 10 to 14 days) treatment with erythropoietin and G-CSF or GM-CSF does not appear to increase the progression to acute leukemia. Patients with low baseline EPO levels appear to fare the best. A study assessing the potential role of darbopoietin (Aranesp) in low-risk MDS began in late 2004. Cyclosporine, an immunosuppressant which we discuss in Chapter 9, has recently been noted to be effective in a rare subtype, hypoplastic MDS.

Thalidomide (Thalomid) which has both anti-angiogenesis and tumor necrosis factor inhibitory properties has modest activity for patients with low-risk MDS. Its dose-limiting toxicity has been neurotoxicity. Lenalidomide is considerably more potent than thalidomide and also does not appear to have the neurotoxic component. Arsenic trioxide (Trisenox) also has activity in both low- and high-risk MDS. It works by inducing apoptosis and suppressing leukemia progenitor proliferation. Other novel agents in clinical trials for MDS include the monoclonal antibody that neutralizes the vascular endothelial growth factor receptor, bevacizumab (Avastin), which was recently approved by the FDA for the treatment of metastatic colon cancer.

Lymphomas

Hodgkin lymphoma

Early-stage Hodgkin lymphoma

Up until about 10 years ago, there was reasonable agreement that for patients with early-stage or the localized form of HL (stage I or II), an extended field (a field that encompasses all lymph node sites either above or below the diaphragm) radiotherapy was effective treatment (Figure 7.6). However, studies have shown that although most patients (95%) achieve a complete remission, almost a quarter of these patients are at risk of subsequent relapse. This paved the way towards treating some patients with early-stage disease with some chemotherapy. Currently most specialists advocate extended field radiotherapy alone for patients with early-stage disease who have 'non-bulk' (defined as less than 10 cm in greatest diameter) and stage IA epitrochlear or high-neck disease; patients with the distinct subtype, lymphocyte-predominant can be treated with involved field (involved node groups with a small margin of adjacent normal tissue) radiotherapy only. There is, however, no significant difference in overall survival between those treated with chemotherapy for recurrence (following initial radiotherapy) and those who received chemotherapy initially. There are other factors, such as the psycho-

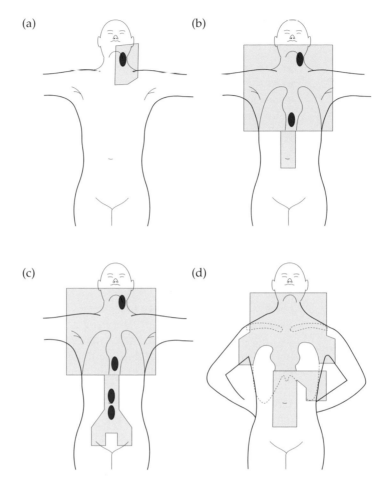

Figure 7.6   A schematic representation of (a) involved field, (b) extended field, (c) total-nodal irradiation, (d) mantle plus upper abdomen radiotherapy treatment for patients with Hodgkin lymphoma.

logical effects of treatment failure and further treatment, which will often be extended (as for the treatment of advanced disease; see below), and the long-term effects. It is therefore important for the specialist to discuss the different treatment strategies and tailor the therapy to the individual patient. When chemotherapy is used, the combination ABVD (adriamycin or daunorubicin, bleomycin, vinblastine and dacarbazine) is often the preferred treatment. This has been shown to be effective and appears to have the potential for reducing long-term side-effects. Currently four 'cycles' or courses of ABVD have been formally tested, but even briefer chemotherapy and/or reduced doses of radiotherapy are being tested. Most specialists, therefore, offer the majority of patients with early-stage disease, four cycles of ABVD chemotherapy followed by involved field radiotherapy. Patients who are not able to receive chemotherapy can be treated with radiotherapy alone.

The immediate side-effects of chemotherapy are considerably greater than radiotherapy. The combination causes nausea and vomiting, which can occasionally be severe, and hair loss. Bone marrow suppression is common, but serious infections are uncommon; many patients benefit from treatment with G-CSF. The long-term side-effects of both therapies are discussed in Chapter 10.

Bleomycin is a drug which was originally extracted from the fungus *Streptomyces verticillus* from culture broths obtained from soil from a Japanese coal mine. It works by producing single- and double-strand DNA breaks. It can be administered intravenously or intramuscularly, but a test dose is usually given first, since allergic reactions can occur. The principal side-effect is lung toxicity (*pulmonary fibrosis*), which can be much worse in smokers and appears to be related to large doses of the drug. This can result in the lungs becoming stiff and reversal can take months (Figure 7.7). Specialists might monitor the lungs' capacity (pulmonary function studies) once they feel that the cumulative dose is high. The drug can also cause fevers, hair loss, arthritis and skin changes, with many patients noticing a darkening of the skin, particularly around the hands and joints; darkening of the skin can also occur in areas of previous radiotherapy or surgery. These effects are also reversible.

Vinblastine, like vincristine which we discussed above, is a member of the natural vinca alkaloids, which are extracted from the periwinkle plant. Like vincristine, it works by disrupting the microtubules that contain the mitotic spindles within the cell and is given by intravenous injection. Unlike vincristine, its side-effects are mainly related to bone marrow suppression, resulting in moderately severe neutropenia and sometimes anemia and low

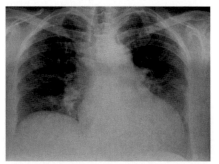

Figure 7.7   A chest radiograph showing lung (pulmonary) fibrosis from bleomycin in a patient with Hodgkin lymphoma (courtesy of Dr John Baird).

platelet counts. Patients receiving this drug should not receive an antibiotic called erythromycin owing to possible severe liver toxic effects; all other antibiotics appear to be safe.

Dacarbazine is an alkylating agent which works by interfering with the DNA synthesis. It is administered intravenously. It can cause nausea and sometimes vomiting; specialists will prescribe the strongest anti-emetics when using this drug. It also causes bone marrow suppression and rarely can be toxic to the liver. The drug is unstable on exposure to light and must, therefore, be covered appropriately whilst being administered.

Advanced stage Hodgkin lymphoma

Patients with advanced disease are those who present with B symptoms or stage III or IV disease. Such patients can be effectively treated with chemotherapy, usually six to eight cycles of ABVD. Over 80% of patients will achieve a complete remission, which is long term for about two-thirds. Patients who have 'bulk' disease (greater than 10 cm in diameter) should receive radiotherapy to these sites (only), once chemotherapy is completed and a complete remission confirmed. Patients also receive radiotherapy if they do not achieve a complete remission or have a minor response to chemotherapy. In view of the increased risk of potential serious late-effects, in particular when a combination of chemotherapy and radiotherapy are employed, every effort is taken to ensure its necessity (Chapter 10).

Many efforts are currently devoted to improving on the results achieved by treatment with ABVD, which has been a significant advance from the historical treatment with MOPP [mechlorethamine (nitrogen mustard), vincristine, procarbazine and prednisone], introduced in 1964. Newer combinations such as the seven-drug combination known as Stanford V (mechlorethamine, daunorubicin, vinblastine, vincristine, bleomycin, etoposide and prednisolone), developed at Stanford, California and the BEACOPP regimen (bleomycin, etoposide, daunorubicin, cyclophosphamide, vincristine, procarbazine and prednisone), developed by the German Hodgkin Lymphoma Study Group, have resulted in better results, particularly in high-risk patients, and further studies are in progress. One of the major concerns with the BEACOPP regimen has been the increased risk of patients to develop treatment-related (secondary) leukemia.

Hodgkin lymphoma in pregnancy

Since HL frequently occurs in young adults, occasionally the diagnosis is made whilst the patient is pregnant. Studies have confirmed that it is quite safe to treat such patients with chemotherapy after the first trimester of the pregnancy. The risks associated with chemotherapy to the fetus are quite small and mainly in the first trimester (first 14 weeks of pregnancy). Specialists will delay chemotherapy until the pregnancy has progressed to the second trimester; alternatively some may discuss the possibility of terminating the pregnancy, if the patient wishes. Radiotherapy is best avoided throughout the pregnancy, in particular abdominal and pelvic radiotherapy, which will harm the fetus (leukemogenicity). When chemotherapy is used, the specialist will bear in mind the side-effects associated, which may affect the fetus in a manner similar to the mother.

Refractory or relapsed Hodgkin lymphoma

Sadly up to a third of all patients with HL will require further therapy at some time for recurrent disease. The efficacy of further chemotherapy or radiotherapy depends upon a number of factors, particularly the duration of remission, the extent of disease at the time of recurrence, advanced age, presence of B symptoms and the choice of initial therapy. Patients who relapse following radiotherapy alone fare well with chemotherapy such as ABVD (as discussed above). Patients who fail to enter an initial complete remission or relapse within a year of completing therapy have a poor prognosis with further conventional chemotherapy and should be considered for high-dose chemotherapy and stem cell transplant. Successful remission can often be achieved, with the same chemotherapy, in about half of the patients who relapse after having been in continuous complete remission for a year or longer.

Rarely a patient may relapse with localized disease after initial chemotherapy. Such a patient can be treated initially with involved field radiotherapy with an excellent chance of long-term remission. In the few patients who cannot achieve a remission, palliative strategies can be used to control symptoms, particularly B symptoms, for long periods of time. Prednisone and drugs such as etoposide (by mouth) are quite useful in this context.

Non-Hodgkin lymphoma

Low-grade lymphomas

Follicular lymphoma

Most patients present with indolent disease (also known as grade 1 follicular lymphoma), which has the least number of large cells and treatment in general has not been shown to result in long-term complete remissions. Many specialists, therefore, may simply observe them carefully and offer no specific therapy. When therapy is indicated, often with the emergence of B symptoms, or increasing disease bulk, single agent chlorambucil has been the historical choice. Combination chemotherapy with anthracyclines, such as CHOP (cyclophosphamide, daunorubicin, vincristine and prednisone), or without an anthracycline, such as CVP (cyclophosphamide, vincristine and prednisone), causes a more rapid response and a higher proportion of complete remissions, though the overall survival of about 8 to 10 years is similar; most remissions last for about 3 years.

Studies assessing the role of immunotherapy, particularly interferon (IFN-α), with CHOP have suggested an improved overall survival with IFN-α maintenance therapy; other studies have confirmed longer remissions but no improvement in overall survival. Newer drug combinations, such as FMD (fludarabine, mitoxantrone and dexamethasone) offer high response rates but are associated with increased risk of potentially serious infections. In some patients treated with FMD chemotherapy, molecular remissions have been observed (loss of the BCL-2 gene rearrangement, which is overexpressed in many patients with follicular lymphoma), but its effect on overall survival has not been proven as yet. Other novel strategies, such as, assessing the role of a protein molecule, called antisense BCL-2 (Oblimersen; Genasense), to reduce the expression of this molecular marker, are being pursued. Very recently, investigators also observed that antisense BCL-2 therapy enhances the antilymphoma activity of another drug, bortezomib (Velcade), showing promising results in follicular and mantle cell lymphomas. About 10 to 15% of patients present with localized disease and can often achieve long-term remission with radiotherapy alone.

Since the majority of the lymphoma cells in patients with follicular lymphoma express the CD20 antigen, the monoclonal antibody rituximab has been extensively studied. In studies of previously treated patients, it has shown a level of activity similar to CHOP, with responses in about 50% of patients, based upon which the drug was approved by the FDA in 1998. Studies assessing its role as a maintenance therapy and also first-line therapy are in progress. It might also be useful as a 'purging' agent for patients receiving an autologous stem cell transplant (Chapter 9). Other monoclonal antibodies, such as tositumomab (iodine-131 conjugated antibody; Bexxar) and ibritumomab tiuxetan (yttrium-90 conjugated antibody; Zevalin) are used as a mean of targeting a therapeutic dose of radiation to the lymphoma cells, by linking them to radioisotopes. Both Bexxar and Zevalin are directed against CD20, but probably against different epitopes from rituximab. Response rates with both agents have been very encouraging and both products are now licensed for use in the treatment of patients with relapsed disease, in the US and other parts of the world, but not yet in the UK.

Toxicity associated with these treatments has been quite low, but persistent low blood counts as a result of bone marrow damage can be a problem with tositumomab and ibritumomab, but not rituximab. In a randomized study comparing ibritumomab with rituximab for the treatment of patients with refractory or relapsed follicular lymphoma, ibritumomab was found to be superior. The side-effects of these treatments are mild and include cough, nausea and occasionally spasm of the airways (bronchospasm). Bone marrow suppression is seen more often in patients receiving ibritumomab and current treatment guidelines suggest it not to be used in patients with more than 25% involvement of bone marrow by lymphoma.

Another area of great interest is the potential to produce an individual vaccine for patients with follicular lymphoma. Landmark studies in the early 1990s confirmed the safety of DNA vaccines in humans and clinical trials of a DNA vaccine containing genes against the malaria parasite began thereafter. Preliminary results confirmed its safety and regulatory bodies in the US and UK, and now some other European countries, approved trials to vaccinate patients with follicular lymphoma in the first instance. A lymph node is removed for DNA extraction and a vaccine is prepared for that particular patient, whilst he/she is subjected to conventional chemotherapy in order to achieve a remission (Figure 7.8 summarizes the vaccination strategy). Once remission is achieved, patients are then vaccinated and followed carefully. No results of note are currently available from these studies which began in 1997. Preliminary results from a related study in which patients were subjected to high dose chemotherapy appeared promising when reported in 1992, but there has been no further information reported since!

The natural history of follicular lymphoma involves an ultimate transformation to a diffuse large cell B-cell high grade lymphoma, which should be treated accordingly. The prognosis of transformed follicular lymphoma is worse than *de novo* diffuse large cell lymphoma.

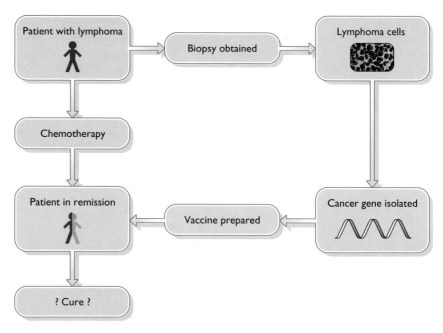

Figure 7.8   A schematic representation of the vaccination strategy for patients with follicular lymphomas.

Mantle cell lymphoma

Mantle cell lymphoma responds poorly to currently available therapies. Anthracycline-based chemotherapy combinations, such as CHOP, lead to a complete remission in less than 50% of all patients, but most of these remissions are short-lived. The average survival from diagnosis is about 3 to 4 years, and those with a high International Prognostic Score fare much worse. Because of this bleak outcome, many patients elect to partake in clinical trials and many younger patients are offered stem cell transplantation. Recently encouraging response rates, which appear durable for at least 2 years (time of analysis), have been reported with an intensive ALL-type chemotherapy, hyper-CVAD in combination with rituximab.

Small lymphocytic lymphoma

Small lymphocytic lymphoma is the tissue manifestation of CLL and the treatment mirrors that of CLL. Most specialists offer therapy only when the patients are symptomatic or have increasing disease bulk. Both chlorambucil and fludarabine are used as first-line therapies, though neither treatment is curative. Histological transformation to diffuse large B-cell lymphoma occurs in about 3% of all patients.

Mycosis fungoides/Sézary syndrome

Patients with mycosis fungoides often present with skin conditions resembling eczema or dermatitis before they begin to ulcerate and it can be many years before a firm diagnosis is made. Those who have circulating characteristic lymphoma cells (Sézary cells) are said to have Sézary syndrome. This skin (cutaneous) lymphoma is incurable with conventional therapy and tends to have an indolent course. Therapies used include topical steroid creams, topical nitrogen mustard, photochemotherapy and a specialized ultraviolet treatment called PUVA (psoralen ultraviolet A-range) therapy. Some patients have had short-term benefit from interferon (IFN-α) (Figure 7.9a and b). Various chemotherapy combinations as well as superficial radiotherapy (electron-beam radiation) have also been used with limited success. Some patients with the localized form of mycosis fungoides can achieve long-lasting remission with radiotherapy.

High-grade lymphomas

Diffuse large B-cell lymphoma

The treatment of patients with diffuse large B-cell lymphoma has met a qualified degree of success since the 1970s, when the CHOP (see above) chemotherapy regimen was introduced. This treatment results in a complete remission rate of about 70%, which are long term for about 40% of the patients. A variety of related chemotherapy regimens and some which are more intensive have now been studied and, though probably equally effective, a meta-analysis confirmed that the CHOP regimen should remain the standard therapy. A recent French study in older patients found that adding

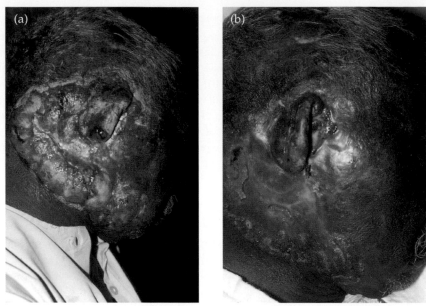

Figure 7.9   A patient with mycosis fungoides treated with interferon alfa: (a) after 3 months and (b) after 6 months.

rituximab to CHOP improved both the disease-free and overall survival and now most specialists consider this to be the standard therapy for older patients. It is of interest that whilst a number of clinical trials are examining this combination in younger patients, some specialists are routinely using this approach and chemo-immunotherapy is becoming the order of the day! In younger patients who present with a high IPI score, it might be reasonable to consider stem cell transplant, once a complete remission is achieved. Approaches aimed at either escalating the doses of CHOP chemotherapy regimen, or administering standard doses on a shortened schedule every two weeks (compared with the conventional 3 weeks), are also being investigated. Since such approaches result in significantly more bone marrow suppression, G-CSF support is essential.

About 60% of all patients will relapse and require further therapy. Patients who relapse from a complete remission can often achieve remission again, with the same treatment, if the previous remission was at least 6 months long. They should then be considered for high-dose chemotherapy and stem cell transplant. Many specialists feel that all patients who relapse within 2 years of completing chemotherapy should be considered for this approach, provided that their disease can still respond to chemotherapy (termed chemo-sensitive). Patients who have chemotherapy-refractory disease tend to fare poorly.

In patients who present with early-stage or localized disease, a brief course of chemotherapy, usually three cycles, followed by radiotherapy will produce long-term remissions in over 80% of patients.

Burkitt's lymphoma

Burkitt's lymphoma can frequently be cured if diagnosed promptly and short courses of intensive chemotherapy regimens, which incorporate high doses of cyclophosphamide, are employed in a timely manner. Since this lymphoma grows very rapidly, tumor lysis syndrome can occur frequently at initiation of therapy and appropriate precautions need to be taken (see Chapter 7). A diagnosis of Burkitt's lymphoma should be considered as a medical emergency and it is best to transfer the patient to a specialist leukemia unit. If the condition is not diagnosed precisely and a CHOP or CHOP-like treatment offered on the basis of a high-grade lymphoma diagnosis, remissions do occur but in general tend to be short-lived. Most specialists use chemotherapy regimens such as CODOX-M/IVAC (cyclophosphamide, vincristine, daunorubicin, methorexate, ifosfamide, etoposide and cytarabine), or similar. Burkitt's lymphoma has a predilection to involve the CNS and so patients should receive 'prophylactic' intrathecal therapy, as in ALL (see above).

Rarely patients with Burkitt's lymphoma present with localized disease, for example involving the small and large bowel junction (*ileocecal* region) where it can be resected completely and has an excellent prognosis with chemotherapy thereafter.

Lymphoblastic lymphoma

Patients with lymphoblastic lymphoma are treated like ALL, often with the hyper-CVAD regimen and CNS prophylaxis therapy. Most specialists prefer to offer a stem cell transplant to these patients once a complete remission has been achieved and we discuss this in Chapter 9. Many of these patients have a large mediastinal mass at diagnosis and should receive radiotherapy also. The long-term success rates for treating patients with the combination chemotherapy, followed by mediastinal radiotherapy and CNS therapy and then subjecting them to an allogeneic stem cell transplant approach about 40 to 50%. Patients with relapsed or refractory disease tend to fare poorly and often do not respond to chemotherapy.

Peripheral T-cell lymphoma

The treatment of peripheral T-cell lymphoma mirrors that of diffuse large cell lymphoma, but most patients tend to do less well and many specialists will consider offering a stem transplant as part of the initial therapy, particularly for the younger patients who present with poor risk features.

Anaplastic large T/null-cell lymphoma

Most patients with anaplastic large T/null-cell lymphoma respond very well to chemotherapy regimens like CHOP, with over 75% of all patients entering a long-term remission (making this one of the most curable forms of lymphoma!) Patients who relapse can often be cured following an autologous stem cell transplant.

Adult T-cell lymphoma/leukemia

Adult T-cell lymphoma/leukemia is sadly, at present, a difficult disease to treat; most patients do not fare well with CHOP-like chemotherapy and the prognosis is poor.

Extranodal lymphomas

Extranodal lymphomas in general are treated as nodal lymphomas, depending on the histological subtypes. Certain extranodal lymphomas, however, present unique management problems which should be addressed accordingly.

MALT (mucosa-associated lymphoid tissue) lymphoma

MALT lymphomas (extranodal marginal zone B-cell lymphoma of MALT-type) at all sites, except the stomach, are in general treated initially as for follicular lymphoma. Since the majority of patients present with localized disease, the treatment often tends to be radiotherapy and over 90% of patients are able to achieve a long-term remission. Patients with disseminated disease respond to chemotherapy, but are rarely curable.

Patients with stomach (gastric) MALT lymphoma are unique since some of them can be cured simply by treating the underlying *Helicobacter pylori* infection, which is causally associated with the lymphoma. If the lymphoma has not invaded the stomach deeply and not transformed into a high-grade large-cell lymphoma, patients should receive the appropriate antibiotics and be followed closely. Eradication of the *Helicobacter pylori* infection results in regression of lymphoma in almost three-quarters of all patients. Non-responding stomach lesions should be treated with simple chemotherapy, such as chlorambucil initially, but radiotherapy or surgical resection may be required for persistent symptomatic disease.

Primary CNS lymphomas

Historically radiotherapy was the treatment of choice for primary CNS lymphomas, but relapses were quite common. Its treatment remains unsatisfactory overall, but encouraging progress appears to have been made with high-dose methotrexate-based chemotherapy regimens combined with radiotherapy. Sadly this combined chemotherapy and radiotherapy approach can result in a number of late neuropsychological side-effects, such as impaired memory and behavioral problems (see Chapter 10). Current studies are assessing the role of chemotherapy alone.

Testicular lymphomas

Testicular lymphomas are usually treated with a CHOP-like chemotherapy regimen, followed by radiotherapy to the contralateral testis and prophylactic intrathecal chemotherapy. With such an approach about 30% of all patients can achieve long-term remission. Studies of adding rituximab to the chemotherapy are in progress.

Myelomas

Multiple myeloma

Patients with mutiple myeloma continue to present a therapeutic challenge and the disease, for the most part, remains incurable. Several new and novel therapies have been introduced over the past decade, and we have a greater understanding of the molecular biology of the disease. The overall survival of most patients with myeloma is around 3 to 4 years. Treatment produces a response in about 70% of all patients, with a fall in the level of paraproteins, a reduction in the number of plasma cells in the bone marrow, a reduction and even resolution of the bone lesions and an improvement, sometimes complete, in the clinical symptoms such as pain. Complete remission, however, as characterized by the complete disappearance of the various criteria which led to the diagnosis is rare, except perhaps with stem cell transplantation, which we discuss in Chapter 9. Post-transplant donor lymphocyte infusions seem to further improve results and more specific cellular therapies, such as therapies with 'natural-killer (NK)' cells and minor histocompatibility-specific T cells, are currently being studied. There is, of course, a significant benefit in the quality of life for most patients.

Specific anti-myeloma therapy usually results in an improvement in the various myeloma parameters, such as the levels of paraprotein, during the course of the disease. These parameters then typically plateau and specialists tend to consider stopping anti-myeloma treatment, as maintenance therapy has generally not been found to be useful. Further therapy, either with the same treatment or a different one, is commenced when the parameters become worse again and the patients often develop symptoms. Eventually patients become refractory/resistant to therapy and develop worsening kidney failure or a life-threatening infection.

Specialists will, therefore, have a structured management plan for most patients with myeloma. Since the majority of patients will have symptomatic disease at the time of the diagnosis, many will require supportive care to control symptoms and also to minimize the risks of myeloma-related complications, such as bone disease and kidney failure, prior to specific anti-myeloma therapy.

Supportive therapy

Pain control is of paramount importance and often requires narcotic drugs and sometimes radiotherapy. Fractures may be present and require surgical fixation at times. Over the past 12 years, specialists have been increasingly using drugs belonging to the bisphosphonate family. Bisphosphonates are drugs which bind to the surface of damaged bones in patients with myeloma and other cancers, and by doing so are able to prevent bone destruction and help in the repair process of bone lesions. They have been found very useful both in the treatment of myeloma-related bone disease and also in controlling bone pain. The most widely used bisphosphonates are pamidronate (Aredia), zoledronic acid (Zometa) and ibandronate (Bondronat), all of which are administered intravenously, and clodronate (Bonefos), which can be given by mouth. Recently an oral preparation of ibandronate (Boniva) has also become available. These drugs work by promoting apoptosis of myeloma cells and the bone cells (osteoclasts). They are potent inhibitors of bone resorption and so inhibit the progression of lytic bone lesions. They also help in the repair of the bone lytic lesions and prevent bone fractures (pathological fractures).

Bone biopsies from patients with myeloma show an unbalanced bone remodeling formation, which on one hand has increased bone resorption and on the other hand lowered bone formation. There is a strong interdependence between myeloma cells and osteoclasts; an increasing number of molecules produced by osteoclasts appear to play a role in the survival and growth of myeloma cells. One such molecule, osteoprotegerin (OPG) produced by osteoclasts has been shown to affect myeloma cell growth. Both pamidronate and zoledronate stimulate OPG production and slow myeloma growth *in vitro* (in the laboratory). Clinical studies have suggested an overall survival benefit from bisphosphonate treatment, confirming their anti-myeloma effects. Bisphosphonates also help control the high blood calcium (hypercalcemia) which can be present. Sometimes specialists may also use steroids and calcitonin, which inhibits bone resorption, to treat hypercalcemia.

A novel drug, currently in clinical trials, AMG 162 (Amgen), is a human monoclonal antibody that works by inhibiting the protein (RANKL) which plays a critical role in excessive bone loss and may have a future role for the treatment of the bone problems associated with myelomas.

In all patients, even those who do not show evidence of kidney failure, it is important to maintain good hydration, with a fluid intake of at least 3 liters per day. Factors which may result in kidney problems, such as hypercalcemia, infection, dehydration and a high level of uric acid, must be sought and treated promptly. Patients who have kidney failure as a result of the myeloma proteins being deposited in the kidneys will require anti-myeloma therapy in addition to kidney supportive measures such as dialysis.

Anemia often results from multiple factors, such as bone marrow infiltration by plasma cells and kidney failure. This usually improves when anti-myeloma therapy begins to work; it can also be improved by blood transfusions and erythropoietins (EPO), such as darbopoietin.

Anti-myeloma therapies

Patients who do not have any symptoms and findings consistent with an indolent or smoldering myeloma often remain stable for long periods and do not require anti-myeloma therapy. Patients with monoclonal gammopathy of unknown significance (MGUS) also do not require any specific therapy. Both categories of patients need to be observed carefully for evidence of disease progression. The development of progressive disease is an indication to commence specific therapy.

In patients who are younger than 70 years of age, most specialists used to favor an aggressive approach with combination chemotherapy using the VAD (vincristine, adriamycin or daunorubicin and dexamethasone) regimen followed by consideration for stem cell transplantation for those who show some response. VAD therapy is administered as a continuous infusion every 3 weeks. This therapy results in over 80% response rates, with about 15 to 20% complete remissions. This is a good choice for patients with kidney failure also, since the drugs are metabolized and excreted by the liver. Studies are currently exploring the use of an oral preparation of idarubicin and dexamethasone, as well as liposomal daunorubicin (Doxil). In patients older than 70 years of age, the preferred chemotherapy is often the historical therapy, oral melphalan and prednisone, first introduced in 1969. It results in an objective response in over half of all patients. Melphalan is a member of the alkylating family of drugs and works by interfering with the protein synthesis of the myeloma cells. At conventional doses, its main side-effects are bone marrow suppression. In high doses it is used as a preparatory regimen for autologous stem cell transplantation and side-effects include severe hair loss, severe nausea and vomiting, profound mucositis, diarrhea and severe bone marrow suppression.

Patients with myeloma respond well to radiotherapy. Local radiotherapy is used to relieve pain and for the treatment of patients who present with spinal cord compression. Total-body irradiation (TBI) is often used as part of high dose chemotherapy preparative regimens for stem cell transplantation.

Interferon alfa (IFN-α) has been shown to have anti-myeloma activity and increases the response rates achieved by chemotherapy. It has also been shown to be of modest value as maintenance therapy, once patients have entered a stable (plateau) phase. It is, however, associated with a number of mild but multiple side-effects (see under CML above), which often worsen the quality of life and make its use less acceptable.

Patients who relapse soon after VAD chemotherapy or are refractory to it can often be treated successfully by thalidomide used either as a single agent or in combination with dexamethasone. The response rates are over 60% for the combination of thalidomide and dexamethasone, with about 15% complete remissions. Recent results from studies in newly diagnosed patients indicate similar rates of response and patients who were subjected to a subsequent stem cell transplant fared well. Most specialists now offer a combination of thalidomide and dexamethasone to newly diagnosed patients.

Thalidomide (Thalidomid) works by reducing angiogenesis but its precise mechanism of action in myeloma is unclear. It is associated with a risk of birth defects and is therefore not used in pregnant patients. It has a number of other significant side-effects, such as neuropathy and increased risk of thrombosis (blood clots), particularly in patients receiving thalidomide and chemotherapy combinations. Specialists often use aspirin as low-dose warfarin (coumadin) to reduce the risk of thrombosis.

Recently many efforts have been directed to a thalidomide analogue,, Lenalidomide (Revlimid). Current results are extremely encouraging in patients who have relapsed following an initial therapy. Lenalidomide has few side-effects, but can cause bone marrow suppression. It is now being investigated as a potential initial therapy and as maintenance therapy post-autologous stem cell transplant.

Bortezomib (Velcade) entered the clinic in May 2003, following its approval by the FDA for use in patients with myeloma who have received at least two lines of therapy and progressed on the last of these. It is now being investigated as a potential first-line therapy and preliminary results show an excellent response rate. These are plans to commence a first-line trial using the combination of bortezomib, thalidomide and dexamethasone. Such an approach should be considerably less toxic than chemotherapy and may improve the subsequent stem cell transplant morbidity. Bortezomib works by inhibiting the proteasome, which results in multiple actions ranging from inhibiting myeloma cell growth to angiogenesis. Other novel strategies currently being pursued in patients with refractory/relapsed myeloma include the use of antisense therapy (oblimersen; Genasense) to overcome drug resistance by inducing apoptosis in chemotherapy-resistant myeloma cells (by down-regulating BCL-2), and arsenic trioxide, which works by inducing apoptosis of drug-resistant myeloma cells and can overcome the anti-apoptotic effects of a cytokine, IL-6, which is a major growth and survival factor for myeloma cells.

Plasmacytomas

Patients with a solitary plasmacytoma of bone are usually treated with localized radiotherapy alone. Studies have confirmed that most patients with this condition are at high risk of a local recurrence and about 50% of such patients develop myeloma over a 15 year period. In about 30% of all patients, an MRI will reveal abnormalities suggestive of myeloma. All patients are therefore monitored carefully for life.

Patients with a solitary extramedullary plasmacytoma, in contrast to solitary plasmacytoma of bone, appear to have a truly localized disease with very few patients relapsing; it rarely progresses to myeloma. Local radiotherapy, rather than surgical removal, is the treatment of choice. In patients with paraprotein, this should be monitored following completion of radiotherapy. In most cases it disappears completely within six months of completing treatment.

Plasma cell leukemia

Patients with plasma cell leukemia have more than 20% circulating plasma cells and are treated as *de novo* plasma cell leukemia when there is no prior history of a myeloma. Most patients fare rather poorly with conventional anti-myeloma therapy. High-dose chemotherapy and stem cell transplant is beneficial with about 20 to 25% long-term remissions. Patients who have a history of prior myeloma have a secondary plasma cell leukemia, which carries a worse prognosis.

Waldenström's macroglobulinemia

The treatment of patients with Waldenström's macroglobulinemia mirrors that of low grade lymphomas. Treatment is often only necessary when patients become symptomatic. Symptoms of hyperviscosity are often treated with prompt plasmapheresis and therapy then often comprises chlorambucil or fludarabine. Combination chemotherapy may result in a more rapid control of the disease, but there is no overall survival advantage. Rituximab has been used to treat patients refractory to chemotherapy with about half responding.

Primary amyloidosis

Patients with primary amyloidosis are often treated with chemotherapy, usually melphalan and prednisone, based largely on the fact that amyloid fibrils consist of a monoclonal light chain which is produced by a clone of plasma cells and, by inhibiting this process, it is possible to reduce the synthesis of the amyloid proteins (and their precursors). This treatment has been shown to improve the overall survival to about 18 months, compared to other therapies, such as colchicines (anti-inflammatory agents), which is about 8.5

months. The overall survival is quite variable, depending on the extent of amyloidosis and the organs affected, for example those with cardiac involvement fare the worst with a survival approaching just 6 months, compared to those with neuropathy, where survival approaches 2 years. It is of note that, though the reduction or elimination of the clone of plasma cells producing the amyloid proteins (also known as an amyloidogenic clone) results in an improvement of the function of an affected organ, it is important to make an early diagnosis before organ damage becomes established.

Almost 50% of patients with primary amyloidosis succumb to cardiac problems. Recent studies with a drug called 4'-iodo-4'-deoxyrubicin (I-DOX) have shown promising results. The drug appears to work by binding to the amyloid fibrils and thereby contributes towards the resolution of amyloid deposits. Preliminary results of high-dose melphalan followed by an autologous stem cell transplant also appear encouraging in patients who do not have significant cardiac involvement by amyloid. Efforts are also being directed towards the development of an immunization strategy against the amyloid proteins.

8

Treatment of leukemias, lymphomas and myelomas and clinical trials: additional considerations

In this chapter we discuss the principal adjunctive or additional therapies used in the management of patients with leukemias, lymphomas or myelomas, to make it easier for patients to tolerate specific anti-cancer therapies or to ensure their administration in a timely manner. We also discuss the role of clinical trials (also called experimental treatments). It is also opportune to emphasize the importance of good hygiene on the part of the patient and staff members, regular hand cleaning and avoidance of contact with infected individuals.

Tumor lysis syndrome

A serious but usually preventable complication can occasionally result from treatment of cancers, in particular hematological cancers. This is termed the tumor lysis syndrome and it may occur spontaneously (i.e. before definitive treatment is commenced) or shortly after therapy has begun. The syndrome is usually due to the rapid destruction (lysis) of cancer cells as a result of treatment, resulting in the liberation of vast quantities of cellular material which overwhelms the filtration system in the kidneys. This leads to a number of biochemical (blood chemistry) abnormalities, such as high levels of potassium, low calcium, high phosphorus, high uric acid and high xanthine (especially in patients treated with allopurinol) and, if left untreated, this syndrome can result in a life-threatening metabolic emergency. Specialists will therefore take appropriate precautions prior to and when treating patients with large tumor burdens (for example those with very high white cell counts, or those with large lymph nodes, such as in Burkitt's lymphoma). Patients at risk of the tumor lysis syndrome must be vigorously hydrated, with appropriate precautions for heart failure (pulmonary edema) before receiving chemotherapy or radiotherapy. Specialists have often treated patients with allopurinol (Aloprim, Zyloric, Zyloprim), a drug which blocks the formation of uric acid by blocking the action of an enzyme called *xanthine oxidase*, but this does carry the risk of xanthine stones and potential kidney damage due to accumulation of xanthine, and, importantly, may take several days to work well. Attempts are made to maintain alkaline urine, but this too has to be monitored carefully since alkalinization increases the risk of phosphate precipitation. Patients with severe renal failure should be treated promptly with renal dialysis, usually hemodialysis.

153

Recently many efforts have been directed to the administration of the enzyme *urate oxidase* as a treatment for the high uric acid. This enzyme is present in many mammalian species, but not in humans. Initially there were many frustrations as there was no widely available therapeutic formulation, but more recently, largely from efforts of scientists at Sanofi Synthelabo, a recombinant formulation of urate oxidase, isolated from *Aspergillus flavus* (and expressed in *Saccharomyces cerevisiae*), known as rasburicase (Elitek; Fasturtec) became available. The same group of scientists had earlier produced a non-recombinant form of urate oxidase (uricozyme), which was found to be very effective, but its use was associated with allergic reactions, often quite serious, in about 4.5% of all patients. Rasburicase has now been evaluated largely in children with leukemias or lymphomas and found to be very effective in reducing the uric acid levels and associated with a significantly lower incidence of allergic reactions. Several large studies are currently assessing the role of rasburicase, in comparison to allopurinol, in the prevention and treatment of tumor lysis syndrome in adults with a variety of hematological cancers and preliminary results appear encouraging.

Drug resistance

Another potentially difficult problem is the emergence of drug resistance. In much the same way as bacteria develop resistance to antibiotics, cancer cells can develop resistance to drugs. The mechanisms involved are usually multiple (Figure 8.1). It is not unusual for blood cancer cells to become resistant by

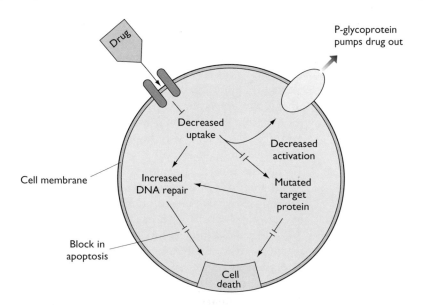

Figure 8.1   A schematic representation of some of the cellular mechanisms for drug resistance.

altering their enzymes. For example, methotexate resistance is associated with alteration of an enzyme (called *dihydrofolate reductase*) which is essential for the activity of this drug. Uniquely, the cancer cell is able to increase the quantity of this enzyme by activating the responsible gene; additionally there is a qualitative alteration of the enzyme. Similarly, resistance can develop to the drug cytarabine by the cell increasing the level of another enzyme (*cytidine deaminase*) which is essential for the action of this drug, and alterations to another enzyme, topoisomerase II results in resistance to the epidophyllotoxins (such as etoposide) and anthracyclines (such as daunorubicin).

Another unique mechanism for drug resistance has been discovered recently. It was observed that when cancer cells are exposed to certain cytotoxic drugs they develop resistance to several other, often unrelated, drugs owing to the alterations to the multidrug resistance (MDR) gene. When the MDR gene is altered, it results in the overproduction of a protein termed P-glycoprotein which confers resistance to the cancer cells by enhancing the cellular elimination of cytotoxic drugs. MDR affects drugs such as the vinca alkaloids (such as vincristine), anthracyclines and epipodophyllotoxins. Researchers have developed a number of novel methods to circumvent this type of drug resistance, for example by treating patients with drugs known as calcium-channel blockers (such as verapamil), often used by cardiologists to treat heart rhythm disorders. Several clinical studies exploring other novel ways of combating MDR are in progress.

Gene microarray studies are being increasingly used to help minimize, and indeed overcome, drug resistance. In August 2004 Amy Holleman and colleagues from Rotterdam (Holland) demonstrated the differential expression of a relatively small number of genes with drug resistance and treatment outcome in childhood acute lymphoblastic leukemias (Figure 8.2). Importantly, they also established that the expression of genes associated with drug resistance has an independent influence on the outcome of treatment of acute lymphoblastic leukemia (Figure 8.3).

Development of resistance to the newer molecularly targeted treatments has also been observed. For example, resistance to imatinib (Glivec; Gleevec) has been increasingly noted in patients with CML, in particular those in the advanced phases of the disease. This resistance appears to result from a variety of diverse mechanisms, including (i) acquired mutations, particularly the so-called 'P-loop' mutations in the Abl kinase domain, which result in structural changes that prevent imatinib binding; (ii) overexpression of the key oncoprotein (P210); and (iii) the production of 'new' proteins which may neutralize imatinib and render it ineffective (Figure 8.4). The emergence of P-loop mutations carries a poor prognosis. It is truly remarkable that leukemia cells have learned to develop resistance over such a short period following the introduction of imatinib into the clinics!

155

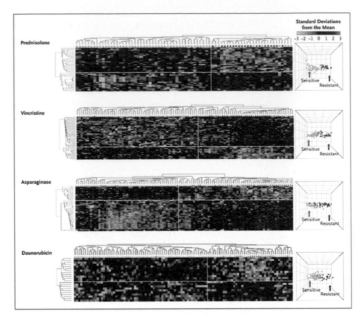

Figure 8.2   Association of genes expressed in children with acute lymphoblastic leukemia and drug resistance [reproduced with permission from Holleman *et al.* (2004) Gene-expression patterns in drug-resistant acute lymphoblastic leukemia cells and response to treatment, *N Engl J Med* 351: 533–42].

Radiotherapy

Radiotherapy (radiation therapy) is another form of intensive treatment used to kill cancer cells by interfering with their growth. Prior to commencing radiotherapy, the radiotherapist (also known as radiation oncologist in the US and clinical oncologist in the UK) must carry out a number of procedures which will enable him/her to localize the area which needs to be treated. He/she will then formulate the treatment plan after discussions with the technical team, who will advise on the selection of the appropriate equipment and calculate the amount of radiation required. It is important to calculate carefully the amount of radiation given because too much is harmful and can even cause cancer (as discussed in Chapter 10). Once the treatment plan has been agreed upon, the technique will be tested (simulated) and then several permanent tattoos will be used to mark indelibly the patient's skin, ensuring that the same areas (volumes) are treated each day.

Normal tissues are often divided into two categories from a radiotherapy perspective: 'acutely responding' implies an immediate reaction during radiotherapy and includes the skin and the lining of the gut; 'late responding' implies that tissues show a reaction many weeks or months following radiotherapy and includes liver, fat, kidney and spinal cord. The effect of a

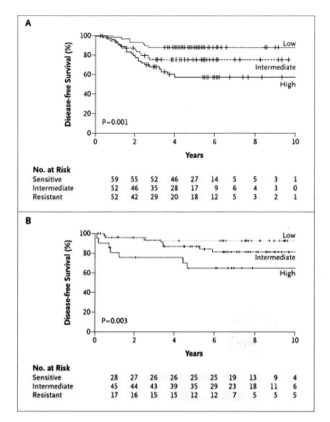

Figure 8.3   Disease-free survival curves according to whether gene expression patterns indicated resistance or not to four drugs used in the treatment of acute lymphoblastic leukemia [reproduced with permission from Holleman et al. (2004) Gene-expression patterns in drug-resistant acute lymphoblastic leukemia cells and response to treatment, *N Engl J Med* 351: 533–42].

part or whole of an organ being irradiated differs according to the tissue concerned. For example, loss of part, or even the whole, of the kidney may lead to very little functional disability, compared with the CNS, where the loss of even a small portion will have serious consequences. Radiotherapy is usually administered by means of a linear accelerator in fractions (sessions) in order to minimize damage to the tissue surrounding the tumor, whilst killing the maximum number of cancer cells (Figure 8.5). The radiotherapist and the technical team will establish the precise dose of radiotherapy per fraction. In general, low dose per fraction is much more likely to spare late effects to normal tissues. When radiotherapy is used as part of CNS therapy, it is usually necessary to divide the treatment over ten fractions (see Chapter 8). Total body irradiation (TBI) is often used in the preparatory regimens for stem cell transplant and is discussed in Chapter 9. In a modern, well-equipped cancer

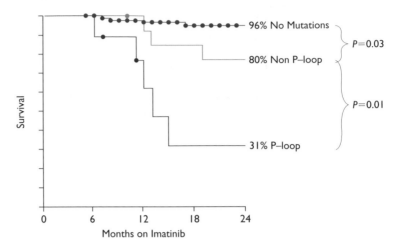

Figure 8.4   Survival curves (Kaplan–Meier) for patients with chronic myeloid leukemia being treated with imatinib who develop resistance owing to mutations [reproduced with permission from Branford *et al.* (2003) Detection of BCR-ABL mutations in patients with CML treated with imatinib is virtually always accompanied by clinical resistance, and mutations in the ATP phosphate-binding loop (P-loop) are associated with a poor prognosis, *Blood* 102: 276–83].

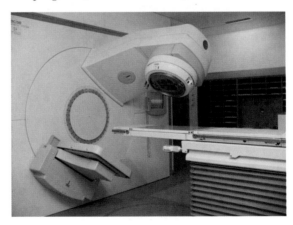

Figure 8.5   A linear accelerator.

center, a whole range of dose fractionation regimens should be available to deal with diverse clinical situations. The biological effect of radiotherapy is not related solely to the total dose delivered, but also to the dose per fraction and the dose rate.

When chemotherapy is combined with radiotherapy in an attempt to increase the cancer cell kill ability, usually there is an enhancement of the effect of radiotherapy on the tissue. Some radiotherapists may also use agents, know as radiosensitizers, in an attempt to increase the targeted effects of radiotherapy on the tumor whilst minimizing damage to surrounding tissue. Various attempts are being made to maximize the radiotherapy effects on the tumor with least toxic effects on the surrounding tissue, for example the volumes of normal tissue irradiated through the use of conformational techniques and intensity-modulated radiotherapy.

Leukapheresis

Leukapheresis is the removal of large numbers of white blood cells from a patient's blood by means of a blood separator (Figure 8.6). This allows the specialist to remove selected cellular components of blood, which is useful for treating patients with leukemias and for collecting particular blood components from healthy blood donors for administration to the patient.

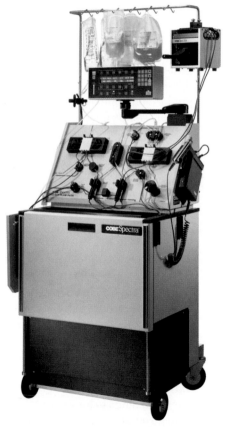

Figure 8.6   A blood cell separator (in this case a Cobe Spectra) (Courtesy of Gambro Laboratories, Denver, Colorado).

159

Leukapheresis is also useful in managing patients with leukemia when chemotherapy cannot be used with safety, such as during the first trimester of pregnancy or an unrelated surgical emergency. It is also useful as an adjunct to chemotherapy in patients whose very high white blood cell counts must be lowered quickly to prevent a major catastrophe such as a stroke, which can result from white blood cells blocking major blood vessels of the brain.

Hemopoietic growth factors

Hemopoietic growth factors (HGFs) are biological agents that help maintain blood production (hemopoiesis) by regulating the proliferation, differentiation and maturation of the hemopoietic stem cells. HGFs play a significant role in the production of cells belonging to all three hemopoietic cell lineages, and a reduction in any of these cell lines results in neutropenia, anemia or thrombocytopenia, respectively. Such cytopenia is commonly witnessed with myelosuppressive cancer treatments. It is possible that appropriate use of HGFs can mitigate these cytopenias.

Myeloid HGFs, such as granulocyte colony-stimulating factor (G-CSF) and granulocyte–macrophage colony-stimulating factor (GM-CSF), and erythroid HGFs, such as erythropoietin (EPO), have been extensively studied in adults and found to be useful in the management of neutropenia and anemia related to both cancer therapy and the cancer itself. HGF use can facilitate the timely administration of cancer treatment and may also improve survival and quality of life (QOL). Currently two preparations of G-CSF are available, filgrastim (Neupogen) and lenograstim (Granocyte). Several preparations of EPO are available, epoetin–alfa (Eprex; Procrit), epoetin beta (NeoRecormon) and darbopoetin alfa (Aranesp).

Significance of neutropenia related to cancer treatments

Cytotoxic chemotherapy can damage the bone marrow integrity, which impairs hemopoiesis and leads to a fall in neutrophil, red blood cell and platelet levels. At conventional doses of chemotherapy, the nadir blood counts are typically observed around day 14 and recovery is complete by day 21 to 28. Most combination chemotherapy regimens have therefore been designed to accommodate the kinetics of bone marrow recovery, which depends upon the stem cell pool is given in 21 or 28 day cycles. The duration and severity of the nadir are clinically significant. When chemotherapy combinations are used at higher doses, the degree and duration of myelosuppression tends to be substantially greater. The greatest risk of infection occurs when the absolute neutrophil count (ANC) falls below 0.5×10^9/liter and remains below this level for more than four days. The risks associated with anemia are greatest when hemoglobin (Hb) levels fall below 8 grams/deciliter (g/dL) and the risk of bleeding is greatest when the platelet count is below 10×10^9/liter.

The severity of neutropenia depends on and is defined by the absolute neutrophil count (ANC) level. Severe neutropenia is defined as ANC $\leq 0.5 \times 10^9$/liter. Though there is no firm agreement of what constitutes febrile neutropenia, most specialists define this as a temperature $>38°C$ in the presence of an ANC of $<0.5 \times 10^9$/liter. The severity and duration of neutropenia is directly related to the risk of infection, which can progress rapidly. Fever is usually the predominant sign of infection and so febrile neutropenia often demands prompt hospitalization and administration of intravenous antibiotics. The mortality rate in cancer patients with febrile neutropenia is about 10%. G-CSF reduces the duration of neutropenia and the incidence of febrile neutropenia in patients treated with cytotoxic chemotherapy. Prophylactic G-CSF reduces the risk of neutropenia and infection-related complications, which in turn reduces the duration of hospitalization and the need for antibiotics. In addition, since the observation that most neutropenic events occur during the first cycle of chemotherapy, some specialists use prophylactic G-CSF from the beginning of such treatments, to help patients receive the planned doses of chemotherapy on time. Several *ad hoc* strategies are employed by specialists to circumvent the problems associated with neutropenia, including chemotherapy dose reduction and treatment delays. Clearly, if the notion of a timely administration of a treatment at specific relative dose intensity (RDI) is important, such a strategy might prove beneficial.

Recent studies assessing the impact of neutropenia on delivery of planned chemotherapy doses in patients with high-grade lymphomas receiving cyclophosphamide, doxorubicin, vincristine and prednisolone (CHOP) chemotherapy have revealed lower response rates and 2-year survival rates in those receiving $\leq 70\%$ RDI compared with patients who received $>70\%$. Studies have been carried out to assess the use of a 'dose-dense' treatment schedule, whereby the conventional doses are administered at shorter intervals in an attempt to improve the overall outcomes. For example, standard dose CHOP administered every 14 days, rather than the conventional 21 days, with prophylactic G-CSF has been shown to improve response and survival rates in elderly patients with lymphomas.

Current treatment guidelines (such as those from the American Society of Clinical Oncology, ASCO) recommend use of G-CSF to prevent neutropenia in patients receiving myelosuppressive chemotherapy with an expected incidence of febrile neutropenia $>40\%$. The possible administration of G-CSF in patients at higher risk of chemotherapy-induced infectious complications is also recommended. Secondary prophylaxis is recommended in patients who have had documented febrile neutropenia in an earlier cycle of chemotherapy or in patients when prolonged neutropenia is causing excessive dose reduction or delay in chemotherapy and for whom chemotherapy dose reduction is not appropriate. Elderly patients may be at greater risk of myelosuppression and the National Comprehensive Cancer Network (NCCN) in the US recommends routine prophylactic use of G-CSF in persons aged 70 years and older, who receive treatment with CHOP or CHOP-like chemotherapy and those aged 60 years and older receiving induction or consolidation chemotherapy for acute myeloid leukemia (AML). The May 2005 NCCN guidelines focus on the assessment of risk for chemotherapy-induced neutropenia and febrile neutropenia, taking into consideration factors such as treatment intent (cure versus palliation), type and dose of chemotherapy agents.

Recently a large European trial assessed the potential role of G-CSF to sensitize (prime) AML cells to cytarabine. Patients were given G-CSF concurrently with cytarabine and idarubicin and another drug called amsacrine given at the end of the treatment cycle (in contrast to the early administration in conventional treatment plans). The specialists noted that although the overall results did not improve, patients with an intermediate-risk stratification appeared to fare better. Further studies are in progress.

The present generation of G-CSF has a short half-life and daily administration, for up to 14 days, is often required. Such frequent injections may dissuade some patients from adherence and increases the burden on healthcare providers. Many efforts have, therefore, been directed to improve on this and one such effort has resulted in the development of a novel molecule, pegfilgrastim (Neulasta). Pegfilgrastim is a sustained duration, pegylated form of G-CSF (filgrastim; Neupogen) that should have the same clinical benefits as filgrastim but require less frequent dosing. Unlike filgrastim, which is primarily excreted via the kidneys, pegfilgrastim is primarily cleared by neutrophils and neutrophil precursors. This 'self-regulating' clearance mechanism results in sustained serum levels of pegfilgrastim for as long as it takes to achieve neutrophil recovery. Hence, pegfilgrastim only requires to be administered once every 21 days. Toxicity analysis confirms that pegfilgrastim can be administered safely; mild-to-moderate bone pain appears to be the only significant adverse event reported so far. Notably, pegfilgrastim was recently approved by the European Medicine Evaluation Agency (EMEA) for the treatment of neutropenia associated with cytotoxic chemotherapy for selected cancers.

Significance of anemia related to cancer and cancer treatment

Although the precise prevalence of anemia in cancer is uncertain, it is generally thought to occur in about 20 to 60% of all cancer patients, with the incidence being the highest for patients afflicted with hematological malignancies. The prevalence, incidence and severity of anemia in the cancer patient depend on several factors (Table 8.1a and b). The age of the patient, the presence or absence of infection, and the presence or absence of concur-

Table 8.1 Prevalence of anemia in cancer	
Breast	20%
Colorectal	15%
Prostate	13%
Ovarian	40%
Myeloma	50%
Non-small cell lung cancer	51%
Lymphoma	60%

rent medical conditions are all important. The histology and stage of the tumor is also important.

Anemia of cancer often develops rather insidiously, and has an impact on virtually all organs and adversely affects a patient's quality of life (QOL). Fatigue is the most common symptom of anemia of cancer and survival of many cancer patients with anemia may be inferior compared with cancer patients without anemia. Anemia is an independent factor in a number of recognized prognostic indices of various hematological malignancies, including CML, CLL, myeloma and Hodgkin lymphoma. It also appears to have a prognostic relevance in lymphoma, but it is noteworthy that currently anemia is not part of the International Prognostic Index (IPI). A French study has confirmed that anemia at diagnosis is indeed an adverse prognostic factor for overall and progression-free survival for most types of lymphomas.

Historically, blood (RBC) transfusion has been the primary mode of treating anemia associated with cancer. RBC transfusions provide a short-term solution but with significant risks such as the potential transmission of infectious agents, including bacteria, viruses, protozoa and prion contamination resulting in Creutzfeldt–Jakob disease (sometimes compared with the 'mad cow disease' in the cow, not in man). Transfusion is also associated with graft-versus-host disease (GvHD), which we discuss in Chapter 9, and results in suppressing the immune system. Over the past two decades, therefore, increasing efforts have been made to use alternative treatments for the anemia of cancer, in particular with recombinant erythropoietin (EPO). The use of these drugs appears to have increased substantially over the past 5 years, as more specialists recognize the full impact of anemia on cancer and its treatments. The recently published guidelines from a joint committee representing the American Societies of Clinical Oncology and Hematology (ASCO and ASH, respectively) recommend the use of EPO for patients with chemotherapy-related anemia with a hemoglobin (Hb) level of less than

10 g/dL. The guidelines also suggested that for selected patients EPO treatment may be indicated for Hb levels of 10–12 g/dL. Similar guidelines are being proposed by national societies in other parts of the world.

A principal drawback of EPO therapy has been the frequent dosing required, which is costly, especially when higher doses are required, and inconvenient for patients (and providers). The new generation of EPO, such as darbopoetin alfa, has a significantly longer half-life and an increased biological activity, which result in increased response rates and a shortened time to response. A number of clinical trials are currently assessing how best to optimize the use of darbopoetin. Studies have confirmed that the time to achieve a target hemoglobin level is achieved faster in darbepoetin alfa-treated patients than epoetin alfa-treated patients. Darbopoetin recently received European and US approval for the treatment of anemia in selected adult cancer patients.

Efforts are also being devoted to develop safe and effective gene therapy directed at erythroid precursors which should facilitate improved methods in the administration of EPO. Katie Binley and colleagues, in Oxford (UK), have developed a gene therapy strategy for the delivery of EPO in a mouse model with a relative EPO deficiency. They demonstrated that long term correction of anemia resulting from erythropoietin deficiency was possible following a single injection of a vector containing a hypoxia-regulated EPO gene. Further studies in larger animals will be required prior to contemplating such studies in humans.

Clinical trials

It should be said that although the treatment of hematological cancers has improved considerably in the past two decades, the overall results are still not entirely satisfactory. It is for this reason that many new treatments are under investigation, and it is often desirable for patients to consider an invitation to participate in a 'clinical trial'. The specialist might offer one or more potentially suitable trials for a patient, but the decision to consider entering a clinical trial or not is always the patient's (or his or her guardian's). Likewise, the patient is completely free to leave a trial at any time, should he or she wish to. Clinical trials are research studies which require careful planning and are designed to determine the value of treatments. There are two important components to them: first, results rather than plausible reasoning by the specialists are mandatory to support the findings of the trial, and second, the trials need to be prospectively planned and are required to provide definitive answers to predefined questions. We are now firmly in the era of evidence-based medicine, as opposed to eminence–based medicine (defined as the practice of medicine based on personal experience and the advice of peers), much of which results from well-designed and ethically conducted clinical trials that lead to proof of safety and efficacy of a particular treatment.

Clinical trials offer potential value to both patients and specialists. They offer the patient variations that may improve on established treatment or, occasionally, a completely new therapy. At the same time, they enable the specialist to evaluate new treatments in an efficient ethical manner. Parenthetically, perhaps it should be mentioned that nearly all advances in cancer treatment have been made through well conducted clinical trials. Clinical trials are carefully controlled and the ethical and legal codes that govern medical practice apply to all clinical trials. The patient (or guardian) must agree to entry into the trial by signing an informed consent form, designed to preserve the patient's autonomy, and the trial itself must first be approved by a supervisory panel, referred to as the Institutional Review Board (IRB), which is made up of individuals who are not involved in the trial itself. The panel will include experts in ethics, scientists, physicians and non-medical (lay) members. There is also a monitoring body, usually a group of specialists in the field who are independent of the trial members, who follow the results and stop a trial if the results of the new regimen prove to be superior to the old, in which case the new regimen will become the standard treatment, or if the results are poorer, in which case the trial will be abandoned.

Some of the largest trials are organized by cooperative groups, linking specialists globally. In the UK, most trials are organized by the Medical Research Council (MRC) and the National Cancer Research Institute (NCRI); in Europe, the largest organization is the European Organization for Research and Treatment of Cancer (EORTC) which brings together a unique European network of over 2000 specialists. In the US, most trials are organized either by the National Institutes of Health (NIH) or by regionally appointed groups (though many operate at a national and often international level), such as the South West Oncology Group (SWOG).

Before any new treatment can be made available, it must be thoroughly tested in the laboratory and in animal studies. If such studies suggest that a particular treatment is safe, then it can be tested in clinical trials, which are carried out in phases, each designed to seek certain information. In the first phase, known as a phase I study, the objective is to determine the best way to give a new treatment and how much of it (dose) can be given safely. Since the emphasis here is not the activity of the drug, patients with different cancers refractory to available treatments are eligible. In contrast, phase II studies require patients with specific cancers to be entered and the emphasis is very much on the anti-cancer effects. Each new phase of a clinical trial depends on the results from the earlier phases. If a treatment is determined to be safe, it enters phase II, and if the treatment shows activity against a specific cancer in phase II, it will enter phase III, when the new treatment will be compared directly with the current standard treatment. Sometimes the specialists will want to incorporate the new treatment into a combination, which is then compared with the standard combination; the combination may include certain types of surgery and/or radiotherapy. Due to the nature of the different phases of the clinical trials, many more patients can anticipate participating in the later phases of the trials.

The results from several large randomized phase III studies are sometimes collated and subjected to stringent mathematical analysis and the results known as a 'meta-analysis'. This methodology is not meant to undermine an individual trial's results, but rather allows the specialists to have a greater degree of confidence that a new treatment or combination is better or worse, when the results of several well-conducted studies are pooled, and able to withstand the intense (additional) scrutiny.

9 *Stem cell transplantation for leukemias, lymphomas and myelomas*

Introduction

Since the early 1920s, specialists have been interested in replacing diseased bone marrow with healthy marrow, not only because the marrow is a source of cancerous cells (although not the only one) but also because the risk of damage to marrow seriously limits cancer therapy. Original observations made by Fabricious-Moeller, in 1922, led to the recognition (in 1949) that lethally irradiated mice and guinea pigs could be protected by the intravenous injection of syngeneic (genetically identical) marrow cells. A few years later, in 1956, Peter Nowell and colleagues demonstrated that the protection from the lethal effects of total body irradiation (TBI) was due to colonization of the recipient by donor cells.

Pari passu many specialists believed that very high doses of chemotherapy drugs would benefit patients with acute leukemias, but it was impossible to give such doses because of the damage caused to normal marrow cells. However, if the patient's marrow, destroyed by TBI or high-dose treatment, could be replaced by new marrow, the amount of drug that could be given would be limited only by its toxicity to other tissues and organs. Extensive experiments in animals showed that this was indeed the case. In addition, it was found that it was not necessary to place healthy donor marrow cells directly into a recipient's marrow cavity – these cells could simply be infused into a vein and they would spontaneously find their way to the marrow cavity where they would begin to grow and reproduce. Successful engraftment depended upon the donor marrow being genetically acceptable by the recipient mouse or the recipient mouse being adequately immunosuppressed. When there was immunological disparity between the mice, and a successful engraftment had occurred, it was observed that following a period of about 2 weeks, the recipient often failed to thrive and developed gastrointestinal and skin problems and later succumbed to infections. This was known as 'runt disease' and we now know this to be the murine equivalent of graft-versus-host disease (GvHD). This research paved the way for bone marrow transplantation in man, largely from the early clinical efforts of Dirk van Bekkum, Robert Good, Georges Mathé, Donnall Thomas and George Santos and their colleagues in the late 1960s and early 1970s. In 1977 Thomas at the Fred Hutchinson Cancer Center, Seattle reported the results of HLA-identical sibling transplants in 100 patients with 'end-stage' leukemia and in 1990 he was awarded the Nobel Prize in medicine for his substantial contributions to this research.

Hemopoietic stem cells

In Chapter 2, we discussed the concept of a single cell (HSC) in the hemo-poietic system which was capable of giving rise to all lineages of the hemo-poietic system for life. This HSC carries an antigen designated CD34, lacks other hemopoietic markers such as CD33, and has no lineage-specific mark-ers. Normal hemopoiesis takes place within the bone marrow, where the HSC and their progeny reside in intimate association with a complex cellular milieu known as the hemopoietic bone marrow environment. Following a stem cell transplantation procedure whereby the donated CD34+ and CD33− cells, which represent about 1×10^3 to 10^4 of the cells of normal hemopoietic marrow, are infused intravenously, hemopoietic cell develop-ment has to be reconstituted within the bone marrow, by a process known as engraftment. It involves a series of complex events, which remain poorly understood. The initial event in the engraftment process, homing, requires a unique recruitment of the infused HSC to the bone marrow, where lodge-ment of the cells then follows. The observation that the HSC were capable of trafficking through the circulation following the intravenous administration, and homing to the appropriate part of the marrow microenvironment was truly remarkable. Once lodged, these HSC accept the environment of the host as 'self' and begin to function! A critical requirement for successful trans-plantation is the availability of sufficient numbers of HSC in the donation (about 3×10^8 'nucleated' cells/kg of the patient's body weight).

Type of stem cell transplant

An allogeneic stem cell transplant is a transplant between two individuals (Figure 9.1). When the individuals are identical twins, the transplant is

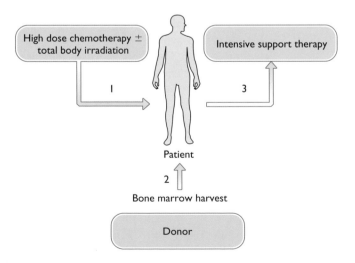

Figure 9.1   A schematic representation of an allogeneic stem cell transplant.

known as syngeneic; when they are not related, the transplant is known as a matched unrelated donor or MUD-SCT. An autologous SCT is a transplant by which a patient's own stem cells are harvested (collected), stored and later returned intravenously (Figure 9.2).

Immunological barriers

In the early stages of stem cell transplantation, since the healthy bone marrow came from a person (host) whose immune and genetic make-up was different from those of the person receiving it (the recipient), serious problems arose from the immunological incompatibility. The ideal donor was therefore an identical twin of the recipient because the genes in both twins are identical and therefore no genetic barriers exist. Transplants between identical twins, syngeneic transplants, were then, and are still, rare. However, subsequent research showed that other family members could also be used, in allogeneic transplants.

In order to understand how non-identical family members can be used as donors, it is useful to look at some of the major immunological barriers to stem cell transplants. These barriers are determined by the major histocompatibility complex (MHC), first described by Jean Dausset in 1958, which

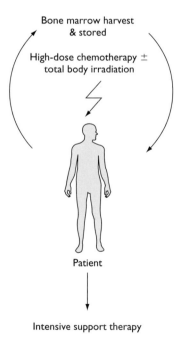

Figure 9.2   A schematic representation of an autologous stem cell transplant.

consists of a cluster of genes located on chromosome number 6 (Figure 9.3). The MHC consists of three classes of genes, known as class I, II and III. The molecules encoded by class I and II are called the human leukocyte antigens (HLA) and these constitute a major component of the immunological barriers. The currently known class I genes are HLA-A, HLA-B and HLA-C and are found on virtually all 'nucleated' cells; class II genes are expressed only on B lymphocytes and a few other cells and the most important genes are HLA-DR, HLA-DQ and HLA-DP. Without going into the fine detail, there is a 25% chance that any one (full) brother or any (full) sister of a patient will have an HLA make-up identical to the patient and therefore be compatible. HLA antigens should not be confused with the major blood group antigens (A, B and O), which are very different. Blood group incompatibility is not a major problem in SCT and, even if it does occur, it is possible simply to centrifuge (spin down) the collected stem cells and remove the incompatible red blood cells. The class III genes include the 'non-HLA genes' which play an important role within the complement (immune) system.

Nowadays most transplant centers carry out the tissue (HLA) typing by molecular techniques, sometimes combined with the traditional serological typing. This is important since the molecular typing can often result in finding rare combinations of genes at the DNA level which might not be expressed on the cell surface and therefore not necessarily important (but some are). Serological tests, on the other hand, detect only antigens which are expressed on the cell surface and therefore miss some antigens which might be important (and will be detected by molecular typing). A combination of these two techniques can often minimize ambiguities between the expressed and not expressed antigens. The World Marrow Donor Association recommends the use of molecular typing for HLA-DR and for HLA-A and HLA-B.

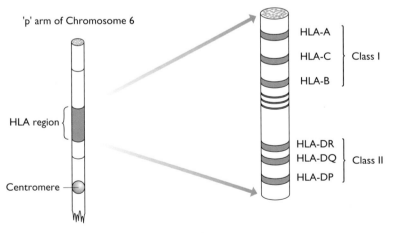

Figure 9.3   The major histocompatibility complex (MHC) located on chromosome 6.

Unfortunately, even when the antigens of the MHC are identical, the acceptance of a stem cell graft is not guaranteed. The donor's T lymphocytes can attack the cells of the host because of minor immunological differences between the donor's and recipient's cells, which are not part of the MHC antigens. These differences can lead to the potentially serious illness of graft-versus-host disease (GvHD). Specialists have developed techniques which can be used to optimize the selection of the best available donor. These include the cytotoxic T-lymphocyte precursor (CTLp) frequency assay which might be a good test to predict the potential for an adverse graft-versus-host reaction. A related test, the helper T-lymphocyte precursor (HTLp) frequency analysis is sometimes useful in determining minor histocompatibility differences between HLA-identical donors, not detected by conventional tests.

Graft rejection by the host may also occur if the recipient's lymphocytes destroy the donor's cells. It is important to distinguish between graft rejection and graft failure. The former implies the recognition and subsequent destruction of stem cells by the recipient's T lymphocytes (and other lymphocytes, known as natural killer or NK cells) and this can often be overcome by immunosuppression. Graft failure, on the other hand, usually implies that the graft has not 'taken'. This could be due, for example, to an insufficient infusion of stem cells or because the donor's marrow is manipulated (treated) with drugs or antibodies resulting in microenvironment abnormalities. Such difficulties are usually non-immunological and will not therefore be corrected by increasing immunosuppression.

These perplexing phenomena led to attempts to suppress the recipient's immune system in order to make rejection and other related complications less likely. A variety of approaches were tried and many were indeed found to improve the success rate of the graft substantially. Most treatment regimens now in use involve chemotherapy, and sometimes radiotherapy, and they are an important part of the bone marrow 'conditioning' programs that establish conditions in which a graft is unlikely to be rejected. A successful conditioning program should also be able to kill any cancer cells which might be present. Most specialists use high doses of the drug cyclophosphamide followed by high-dose radiotherapy to the whole body (TBI), which can be given in a variety of ways. We discuss later how the current ideas on the way an allogeneic SCT works has led to major changes in the conditioning regimens.

Selection of the donor

The success of an allogeneic SCT is substantially reduced with increasing immunological disparity between the donor and the recipient. The best donors are HLA-identical sibling donors because they are not only phenotypically matched for the HLA antigens, but have genotypic identity also.

They are therefore less likely to have problems related to graft rejection and GvHD than to matched unrelated donors, who are only phenotypically matched. Same sex donors are better than mismatched, and for unknown reasons, patients transplanted from male donors fare better than from female donors.

The chances of any one sibling being HLA-identical with the patient are about 25%. It is most unlikely that either of the parents, or the patient's children, will be a complete match since each person inherits one of two possible paternal and one of two possible maternal sets of HLA genes (each set is called a haplotype; see Glossary) to make up the HLA type. In general if the average number of siblings in a family is just over two, the probability of identifying a potential donor is actually about 30%. These constraints obviously limit the number of potential donors considerably. The lack of an HLA identical sibling donor for a patient whose only chance of survival is to have an allogeneic SCT, inspired specialists to try to find acceptable alternative donors, who are not *genetically* HLA identical. These efforts led to establishment of worldwide donor register of HLA-typed individuals, which now include over 9 million HLA-typed volunteers. This pool is currently able to provide suitable donors for about 80% of recipients from a similar racial background. As the number of available donors from diverse racial backgrounds increase, we can anticipate a higher chance of finding a suitable donor.

Graft-versus-host disease (GvHD)

Following an allogeneic SCT, it is important for the newly developing T lymphocytes and the mature T lymphocytes contained in the transplanted cells that recognize the transplant recipient as 'non-self' to be inactivated in order to prevent a GvH reaction. When multiple interactions take place between the donor and host cells, it results in the clinical development of GvH disease (GvHD). The disease was recognized formally in 1966 by Robert Billingham (although the murine equivalent, 'runt disease' had been described a few years earlier). It is mediated by cytotoxic T lymphocytes (CD4+ and CD8+), but the role of specific HLA antigens and minor antigens in determining the attack, and the part played by recipient antigens, has not been worked out in detail. There are two forms of GvHD, acute and chronic, though a clear distinction between them is sometimes difficult. Typically acute GvHD occurs within the first 100 days post-allogeneic SCT. Acute GvHD affects the immune system, liver, skin and gut, but other organs can also sometimes be involved. It produces rashes, severe diarrhea, liver test disturbances, weight loss and, occasionally, serious infections (Figure 9.4). Grades III and IV acute GvHD are an important cause of transplant-related morbidity and mortality.

The incidence of acute GvHD varies from 10 to 90%, depending upon many factors, such as the donor–patient histocompatibility, the sex of the donor,

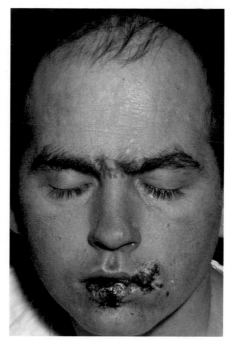

Figure 9.4   A patient with acute graft-versus-host disease involving the skin and lips (courtesy of Prof Rainer Storb).

patient's age, intensity of the conditioning regimen and the type of GvHD prophylaxis. Since acute GvHD is manifested by T lymphocytes, many efforts to deplete these cells from the recepient's harvested cells were attempted. These efforts met a qualified success but the incidence of relapse from disease was extraordinarily high, as discussed later. Today steroids, cyclosporine (a calcineurin inhibitor) and methotrexate remain the mainstay of treatment of acute GvHD. Cyclosporine can produce kidney problems which may result in fluid retention and high blood pressure; it may also produce hair growth over the entire body (hirsutism) and characteristic neurological disabilities, including blindness. These are usually reversible when the drug is stopped. Some specialists favor the agents such as mycophenolate mofetil (MMF, CellCept), anti-thymocyte globulin (ATG), tacrolimus (FK506, Prograf) and rapamycin (Rapamune, sirolimus). More recently a number of specific anti-T-cell monoclonal antibodies have been found to be effective in pilot studies.

Chronic GvHD is a complex, multisystem disease with features of auto-immunity and immunodeficiency which mainly affects the skin (Figure 9.5). It may follow acute GvHD or arise *de novo* 100 days or later post-allogeneic SCT. About 30 to 50% of all allogeneic HLA-matched sibling SCT recipients and about 50 to 70% of unrelated donor bone marrow recipients develop chronic GvHD. The incidence appears to be much higher when the HSC are

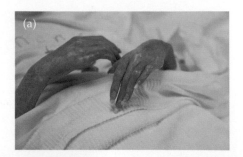

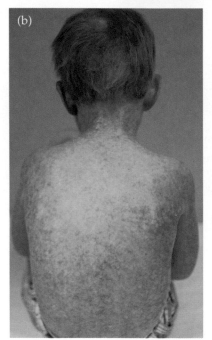
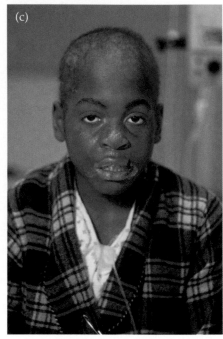

Figure 9.5   A patient with chronic graft versus host disease involving (a) the hands (b) & (c) the skin (courtesy of Prof Rainer Storb).

harvested from peripheral blood rather than the traditional bone marrow, as discussed later. In contrast to the treatment of acute GvHD, which has improved significantly over the past two decades, treatment of chronic GvHD remains difficult and patients with extensive chronic GvHD fare poorly. Conventional therapy is steroids with cyclosporine plus or minus methotrexate; in patients who do not respond to steroids, thalidomide, with or without photopheresis [whereby lymphocytes from the patient are treated with psoralen and ultraviolet A (PUVA) and then transfused back into the patient] have been found to be quite useful.

Graft-versus-tumor (GvT) effect

In 1990 it was established that the immunological attack on normal tissues which produces GvHD was linked to an ability to attack abnormal tissues, particularly cancer, producing a graft-versus-tumor (GvT) effect. The observation that patients with chronic myeloid leukemia (CML) who had allogeneic SCT and developed GvHD had considerably less relapse, though not better overall survival, than patients without GvHD led to the idea that there must be a specific GvT, in this case graft-versus-leukemia (GvL), effect. This was considered to be the first line of evidence for the notion of GvL in CML and the concept derived support from results of syngeneic SCT where no GvHD occurs and relapse rates are very high. Further evidence was collated when attempts to reduce GvHD by depleting T lymphocytes from the harvested stem cells prior to being infused into recipients with CML was found to be remarkably effective, but there was a significant increase in relapse rate of CML. This confirmed the hypothesis that the GvHD effect is accompanied by the GvL effect, and both are dependent on T cells. The efficacy of donor lymphocyte infusions (DLI), which we discuss shortly, lends further support. Much effort, largely from John Barrett and Shimon Slavin, has gone into trying to identify the cells that mediate the GvT effect and to see if they can be separated from those that produce GvHD. It is not yet clear whether the cells responsible for GvT are identical to those which produce GvHD or whether it is a separate population. The problems and disparity only apply in the allogeneic SCT and are absent when autologous stem cells are used to restore hemopoiesis after intensive chemotherapy.

Hemopoietic chimerism

After allogeneic transplantation the recipient's hemopoietic system may be entirely of donor origin (known as donor chimerism), entirely of recipient origin (signifying complete graft rejection followed by an autologous recovery), or a mixture of donor and recipient (host) cells (known as mixed chimerism). The Chimera (a Greek word χίμαιρα), in mythology, was a fire-breathing creature which had the head of a lion, the body of a she-goat and the tail of a dragon. In medicine, the term describes an organism whose body contains cell populations from different individuals of the same or different species occurring either spontaneously or created artificially. Chimerism analysis following an allogeneic transplantation is very useful since the presence of a mixed chimerism often indicates individuals at risk of disease relapse and also helps predict graft rejection.

Sources of hemopoietic stem cells

Bone marrow

From the earliest efforts to offer stem cell transplantation to humans until about 1993, all donations were collected from the bone marrow and this

175

remains a principal source of HSC in allogeneic SCT. Bone marrow is harvested with the patient (for autologous SCT) or the donor (for allogeneic SCT) under general anesthetic by aspiration from the pelvic bones (iliac crests) and, if necessary, the sternum (the breast bone). For a successful graft, about 1 liter of bone marrow is needed, which takes about 90 minutes to collect. In order to prevent the donor from becoming anemic, a blood transfusion may be given during the procedure. Usually the blood transfused is the donor's own blood which was taken about 2 weeks earlier. This is termed an autologous transfusion; it not only avoids unnecessary demands on the blood bank but also, more importantly, avoids the risks, minimal though they are, associated with transfusions from other people, such as transmission of hepatitis or HIV infection.

Peripheral blood

Since 1993, specialists have been increasingly using peripheral blood for harvesting stem cells. HSC may be mobilized into the peripheral blood following administration of G-CSF (see Chapter 8). For allogeneic SCT, donors usually receive G-CSF for about 5 days, following which they usually have a granulocyte count of 30×10^9/liter or more and CD34+ cells appear in the blood, reaching a maximum on the 5th day following G-CSF treatment, which appears to be quite safe for use in healthy people (for purposes of HSC mobilization); there can be some concern if the granulocyte count rises very high. Peripheral blood is then collected by the procedure of blood cell separators, such as the Cobe Spectra, which use automated programs to facilitate efficient collection of CD34+ cells (see Figure 8.6, Chapter 8). Usually an average of 3×10^6 CD34+ cells/kg body weight of the recipient, the amount needed for an HLA-matched sibling allogeneic SCT, can be collected following a single procedure; higher amounts of CD34+ cells, around 10×10^6/kg are required for other types of allogeneic SCT. For autologous SCT, the concentration of CD34+ cells may be increased further by giving the patient cyclophosphamide before starting G-CSF. Sometimes enough CD34+ cells are found in the peripheral blood following recovery from the cyclophosphamide's myelosuppression that G-CSF may not be necessary. Clearly chemotherapy drugs cannot reasonably be used in healthy donors!

Studies have confirmed the success of HSC harvested from peripheral blood and more rapid engraftment than that seen with bone marrow-derived HSC. On the other hand, an increased risk of GvHD, particularly chronic GvHD, has been observed. This is probably related to the increased number of T cells in the peripheral blood donations. Regardless, the ease of collection of the HSC and the rapid engraftment obtained have led many centers to use this for almost all autologous SCT and the use for allogeneic SCT is also increasing.

Umbilical cord

The use of umbilical cord blood-derived HSC has been pioneered by Eliane Gluckman and colleagues in Paris, since 1988. The major drawback has been the quantity of HSC in each cord blood collection; the numbers are usually only adequate to engraft a child recipient. There is also a hypothetical risk of introducing a latent genetic defect which might appear many years after a successful transplant. The major advantages are the abundant supply of umbilical cord blood with no risk to mother or infant, and the immaturity of the immune cells might reduce the risks of immunological disparity and subsequent GvHD. Umbilical cord cells also have a low viral contamination and can be easily frozen and stored for subsequent use. Currently efforts are being directed to increasing the number of stem cells in a given cord blood sample by using medical devices such as the RepliCell System pioneered by Aästrom Biosciences.

Conditioning regimens

Historically the principal objectives for SCT conditioning regimens were immunosuppression (to prevent graft rejection), disease eradication and 'space-making' (it was believed that stem cells must occupy well defined niches within the marrow stroma). It is now clear that stem cells do not occupy prescribed spaces in the marrow and so 'space-making' is not strictly applicable. The objective to eradicate disease was perceived to be the main reason for the success of a transplant: the thinking then was that the conditioning regimen eradicates the disease and makes the space for the new stem cells, which 'rescues' the patient. The concept of graft-versus-tumor (GvT), discussed above, has clearly changed these thoughts.

In the 1980s, much emphasis was placed on intensifying the conditioning in order to eradicate as much of the disease as possible. Although this is important, the toxic effects were profound, involving the gut, kidneys and bladder, lungs and the heart, which accounted for many of the transplant-related deaths. Specialists are constantly striving to make conditioning regimens less toxic, and GvT does allow us to reduce the intensity significantly, but this effect, important as it is, is not present in all diseases and also cannot be responsible for the success seen in autologous and syngeneic stem cell transplants.

Non-myeloablative transplants

The recognition of a GvT effect has led to significant changes in the way allogeneic transplants are carried out. When bone marrow transplantation conditioning regimens were first used to treat hematological cancers, the transplants were intended primarily as a means to reconstitute marrow function after a massive cancer-ablative treatment with 'supralethal' doses of total body irradiation (TBI). Transplantation conditioning regimens are now designed to focus less on the ablative power and more on the establishment of donor immunity to provide a GvT effect: GvL for patients with leukemias, graft-versus-lymphoma for patients with lymphomas and graft-versus-myeloma (GvM) for those with myelomas.

In 1995, this new thinking paved the way to a new form of allogeneic SCT, known variously as mini-allogeneic SCT, non-myeloablative SCT or a low-intensity conditioning allogeneic SCT. The drug fludarabine has become a central component of these conditioning regimens because of its potent immunosuppressive but non-myeloablative action. The decreased toxicity associated with this approach has facilitated a potentially safer application of transplants to older and debilitated patients. However, these regimens often fail to control the disease, and the search for safe anti-cancer agents to combine with fludarabine has continued. One such example, for patients with leukemias, is the combination of fludarabine and busulfan, which appears to be not only more effective anti-leukemic therapy but also less toxic than TBI. Further attempts to improve on this combination include adding agents which could enhance the GvL effect. Similar searches are ongoing for patients with lymphomas, particularly low-grade lymphomas, and myelomas.

An immediate spin-off of this technology has been the potential application of a GvM effect for patients with myeloma being subjected to autologous transplantation. Efforts are being directed to treat patients with myeloma with conventional high-dose chemotherapy (melphalan) and autologous SCT, followed about 100 days later by a reduced-intensity allogeneic SCT for the cohort with a suitably matched donor.

The major challenges with reduced-intensity allogeneic SCT have been disease eradication, engraftment and GvHD. A modified technique for patients with CML, AML and myelomas, which allows for a more intense conditioning (a midi allogeneic transplant), is now being tested. This may produce adequate disease control to allow time for establishment of a GvL or GvM effect, respectively, as well as allowing engraftment of CD34+ stem cells, which may not engraft with less-intensive reduced-intensity regimens. The objective would be to offer an allogeneic SCT with results similar to a conventional SCT but with lesser side-effects and fewer failures.

Donor lymphocyte infusions

Work carried out by Hans Kolb and colleagues in Munich, in 1990, showed that patients with CML who relapse following an allo-SCT could achieve a subsequent remission simply by receiving donor lymphocyte infusions (DLI). They and others attributed these complete molecular remissions (absence of molecular evidence of disease) to a GvL effect. Many efforts have now established a definitive role of DLI following an early relapse in patients with CML, AML, MDS and myeloma; the technology has met less success in ALL and lymphomas, so far. DLI has also been used successfully to induce remission in patients who fail to eradicate all evidence of disease following a reduced-intensity allogeneic transplant.

Management of patients undergoing stem cell transplantation

What happens to the donor?

For a bone marrow-derived HSC donation, the donor will require a general anesthetic and might have some discomfort or pain at the sites of bone marrow aspiration. The HSC collection is fairly rapid and most donors only need about two days in hospital. For peripheral blood HSC donation, they need a greater degree of involvement, with daily G-CSF injections followed by a day spent in the apheresis unit. The donor suffers no permanent loss of marrow function, since the bone marrow regenerates fully in a few weeks.

Psychological effects pertaining to the donation are, however, not uncommon. Some donors feel guilty if the recipient does not fare well following the SCT; others may feel rejected if initial tests suggest that they may be potential donors but subsequent tests identify a more suitable donor within the family. It is important for all donors to realize that the success or failure of SCT is totally unrelated to recognizable characteristics of the donor.

What happens to the recipient?

There has been a major shift over the past decade in the transplant care from a hospital setting to ambulatory facilities, and indeed in some cases to an outpatient setting. This has been made possible owing to a number of factors, particularly the availability of hemopoietic growth factors such as G-CSF, better support with blood products and antibiotics, and less toxic ways of controlling rejection and GvHD, as well as better selection of recipients and improved tissue typing. Most autologous and some reduced-intensity allogeneic SCT can now be carried out in specialized ambulatory facilities, outpatient departments and even patients' homes. The majority of patients receiving conventional allogeneic SCT require hospitalization for about 4 weeks, some of which is spent in isolation rooms, ranging from those with laminar air flow to ordinary clean rooms, to minimize the risks of infection (Figure 9.6). It has been difficult to prove that any one form of isolation is better than another. Moreover, excellent results can now be obtained without protective isolation facilities. It is possible that control of room air quality through filtration might be important to reduce transmission of fungal spores such as aspergillus. Regardless of the precise venue selected for the individual patient, his or her care requires an infrastructure and organization for multidisciplinary care provided by personnel experienced in the field transplantation and includes specialists, physicians, nurses, house staff (junior medical staff), pharmacists, dieticians, social workers, psychologists and

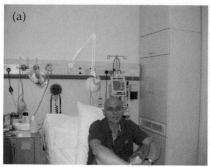 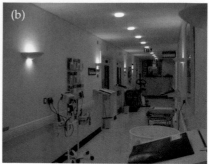

Figure 9.6   An isolation room (a) and the adjacent corridor (b) at the Sir John Dacie Stem Cell Transplant Unit, Hammersmith Hospital at Imperial College, London, UK.

technical support staff. All transplant centers are able to collect data, maintain patient records accurately and exchange scientific information with other centers. Since 1997 a formal audit process has been in place for all member centers of the EBMT and similar initiatives are taking place for members of the CIBMTR.

In most centers, patients for a conventional allogeneic SCT will be admitted about 10 days before the actual transplant. Following a thorough examination, a catheter, usually Hickman catheter, is inserted to provide easy access to circulation. The patient is then commenced on a conditioning regimen designed to eradicate residual cancer cells and to induce immunosuppression in order to minimize the chances of the graft being rejected. Conditioning is followed by infusion of the donor HSC, after which the technical aspects of the SCT procedure are complete and the supportive phase begins.

Following an allogeneic transplant, all patients stay in isolation rooms and some need intensive nursing care for the first 15 to 22 days. As a direct result of the conditioning procedure, patients develop a marked reduction in all of their blood cells (pancytopenia) which lasts about 20 days, until the donor HSC have grown (engrafted) and begun to produce blood cells. During this period of pancytopenia, the patient is at high risk for infection and will also have anemia and thrombocytopenia which will necessitate red blood cell and platelet transfusions; all blood products must be irradiated in order to destroy the allogeneic T lymphocytes which could otherwise generate lethal GvHD. The remaining blood cells are not damaged by this irradiation.

To safeguard against infections, all allogeneic transplant recipients receive intravenous antibiotics which are effective against a wide range of organisms, as well as antiviral, such as acyclovir and famciclovir, and antifungal agents, such as fluconozole, given by mouth during the period of pancytopenia. Occasionally, intravenous antifungal drugs such as voriconazole

(Vfend) and liposomal amphotericin-B (Ambisome) will also be required to prevent serious fungal infection. Many centers also advocate the use of G-CSF to hasten the production of white cells during this period. The spectrum of infectious complications seen during this post-allogeneic transplant period varies in accordance to the time scale. During the first 30 days following a transplant, the primary immune defects are from the low white cell count, breaches in the skin/mucosa barrier and acute GvHD, and bacterial infections and (invasive) fungal infections, such as aspergillus and candida (yeast), predominate. Between 30 and 100 days after transplant, the principal immune defect is an impaired cell immunity as well as mucositis and acute GvHD and there is an increased incidence of viral infections, particularly cytomegalovirus (CMV) infection. After 100 days following an allogeneic transplant, both cellular and humoral immunity is defective and patients may have chronic GvHD. During this period there is an increased risk from 'opportunistic' infections from bacteria, fungi and from viral reactivation, such as chicken pox and herpes simplex.

In general patients subjected to autologous SCT do not have such a high risk of infectious complications and their period of low white cell count is also considerably less; but they do experience problems related to GvHD. Patients who undergo reduced-intensity allogeneic SCT fare somewhere in between the autologous and the conventional allogeneic SCT, with regards to such complications.

During the first 10 days following any type of transplant, most patients develop mouth ulcers (sores), which can be quite debilitating. Many experience pain requiring intravenous narcotics and special nutritional care is needed. Good nutrition is critical since malnutrition is itself immunosuppressive. Specific measures to prevent these serious mouth problems have not been established, but clinical trials are assessing the potential roles of keratinocyte growth factor (KGF; Palifermin) and glutamine. Good dental and oral hygiene is critical for all SCT candidates (and everybody in general). Sometimes drugs like pilocarpine (Salagen) help with the dry mouth. Most patients lose weight, have a reduced calorie intake and become anorexic and require supplemental nutrition. During the transplant period, dieticians try to ensure diets of 2000 to 3000 calories a day, consisting of freshly cooked foods containing few bacteria. In addition, the majority of patients need intravenous parenteral feeding (TPN), particularly where gut GvHD is present.

It is not uncommon at this stage to encounter psychological problems ranging from anxiety related to the transplant procedure and lack of social contact while in isolation, to severe claustrophobia and dependency. To minimize these effects, social contact is allowed during the isolation period as long as it complies with the rules of reverse barrier nursing. This requires the visitors (as well as the medical staff) to be 'isolated' from the patient by wearing a gown, gloves, face mask and a hat when in contact. This is done in order to reduce the chances of the patient acquiring an infection. Most partners and parents want, and are given, unlimited access to a patient's room. Food should ideally be cooked to destroy bacteria; food frequently contaminated with bacteria, such as soft cheeses, soft-boiled eggs, salami and other cold cuts of meat, salads and live yoghurt, are avoided and only peeled fruits are allowed.

The post-transplant period involves considerable disruption and often requires the entire family to change its lifestyle. However, the difficulties are much more acceptable when the outcome is successful. Most transplant centers encourage the patient and a member of his or her family or a partner to stay near the center for about 6 months following an allogeneic SCT and about 2 months following an autologous SCT.

Towards the end of the first month after transplant, most patients are in good condition, with blood counts approaching normal, and they are allowed to leave the hospital. However, their immune system remains defective and will not return to normal for up to 2 years. It is therefore important for the continued success of the transplant to maintain very close medical follow-up of all patients, usually with weekly or fortnightly outpatient visits for the first 6 months.

The most serious complications which may arise during the 6 months after allogeneic transplant are lung inflammation (interstitial pneumonitis) and GvHD. The lung condition is a result of the combined effects of GvHD, previous chemotherapy, radiotherapy given as part of the conditioning regimen, and viral infections; a history of cigarette smoking probably contributes to this. One particular viral infection, due to cytomegalovirus (CMV), is especially important. Currently, there is no totally reliable treatment to prevent CMV infection, but ganciclovir can be effective in suppressing or eradicating CMV infection, though, interestingly, it does not improve survival; recently an oral form of this drug, valganciclovir (Valcyte) has entered the clinics. The overall incidence of lung inflammation is 5 to 20% and, sadly, most of the patients who acquire this will die. Antiviral prophylaxis probably does not work in preventing CMV infections. Rarely lung inflammation is seen following an autologous transplant, but it is often easier to manage since the immunosuppression is less profound and less prolonged than that which occurs with an allogeneic transplant.

By the end of the 6 month period following SCT the majority of successfully transplanted patients are able to resume most of their normal day-to-day activities. They are usually seen at their local hospital/clinic about once a fortnight for a month and monthly thereafter for a year; they are also seen at the transplant center about 3 to 4 times a year. After about 2 years, when the immune system is expected to have recovered, a program of re-immunization with inert or killed vaccines (live vaccines must never be given to a SCT recipient) can be started safely. This is important because all previously donor acquired immunity will be destroyed by the transplant procedure.

Unfortunately relapse is a serious problem in all types of hematological cancers, most often within the first 2 years after the transplant. However, after this, the risk gradually decreases to become minimal after about 5 years, with the major exception of patients with CML who may relapse after many years of leukemia-free survival. This is in keeping with the natural history of CML and its slow evolution (see Chapter 4). Patients with most other hematological cancers can be confidently assumed to be cured after 8 years of being disease free; in CML relapses are rare after 10 years of being disease free. The risk of relapse following transplant for AML seems to be higher in people older than 40 years of age and in those with poor prognostic features such as a high white cell count at the time of diagnosis.

Most patients who survive for 5 years or more following a SCT enjoy normal health and are able to pursue a lifestyle which they enjoyed prior to being diagnosed. Data from both the CIBMTR and the EBMT of patients who had been transplanted and were disease free at 5 years suggest that whilst over 90% of all patients had a productive and good-quality life, some still faced the prospects of illness and even death. The chief causes of death were relapse (late) of their disease, development of a second cancer and chronic GvHD. We discuss the problems of a second cancer related to cancer therapy in Chapter 10.

Clinical results of stem cell transplantation for leukemias

Acute myeloid leukemia (AML)

Allogeneic stem cell transplantation for AML

Allogeneic SCT from an HLA-matched sibling donor has been standard treatment for acute myeloid leukemia (AML) in first complete remission for two decades. It offers a 50–60% chance of long-term remission and possible cure; the risk of relapse is 20%. This reduced relapse rate is largely due to the GvL effect of the allograft against residual leukemia cells. The toxicity of the procedure and mortality owing to transplant-related complications, such as immunosuppression and GvHD, account for 20 to 25%. There have been no prospective randomized trials of allogeneic SCT, but comparative analysis of patients with suitable donors versus those without such donors has confirmed the survival benefits conferred by allogeneic SCT in first complete remission. In recent years results from intensive chemotherapy have improved (as discussed in Chapter 8) and there has been a better stratification of patients' risk of relapse. Allogeneic SCT remains the only potentially curative treatment for patients with AML who fail to respond to induction therapy. The use of reduced-intensity SCT has raised the age limit to 70 years, and possibly higher!

Allogeneic SCT has no role in the management of acute promyelocytic leukemia (APL) in first remission since the results from current induction treatments are excellent. There are, however, no studies that have compared the results of SCT in relation to the induction therapy containing ATRA. Registry data (EBMT) on patients with APL treated in the pre-ATRA era, who received SCT in first complete remission, suggested that 45% of such patients had long-term remissions and possible cure. Allogeneic SCT may be useful for patients who relapse following an arsenic trioxide (Trisenox)-induced second complete remission.

Autologous transplantation for AML

Autologous SCT has also been widely used for the past two decades and current data collated by the EBMT suggest a long-term survival rate, and possible cure, of 45–55%. Relapse is the most common reason for failure, possibly because of residual disease and the loss of a putative GvL effect in the autologous transplant procedure. This is offset by the appreciably lower risk of transplant-related mortality, but it is noteworthy that 5–8% of patients die in complete remission often because of poor engraftment. There is no evidence that purging (*in vitro*) of the harvested stem cells confers additional benefit. A UK-MRC-AML trial assessed the value of adding autologous SCT to a cohort of patients who had already received intensive consolidation (post-remission) therapy. This trial showed a substantial reduction in risk of relapse with autologous SCT resulting in a superior 7 year progression-free survival, despite a higher mortality rate in the transplantation group. A US trial comparing chemotherapy (high-dose cytarabine) with autologous or allogeneic SCT during first remission of AML showed an equivalent event-free survival and a better overall survival with chemotherapy than autologous or allogeneic SCT. A number of other global trials are currently in progress and should help define the role of autologous SCT in AML better.

Acute lymphoblastic leukemia (ALL)

Allogeneic transplantation for ALL

Allogeneic SCT using an HLA-matched sibling donor is often offered to patients with acute lymphoblastic leukemia (ALL) who have failed remission induction or have achieved a second complete remission. Transplantation in first complete remission, as consolidation therapy, is considered unproven at present but may well be the desired treatment for those patients who fall in the poor-risk category. Patients who have Ph-positive (BCR/ABL positive) ALL, have a high white blood cell count at diagnosis, the Burkitt's morphology (FAB subtype L3), certain other cytogenetic abnormalities, such as t(4;11) and t(1;9), or fail to respond to conventional therapy are all potential candidates for an allogeneic SCT in first remission and are able to achieve a 5-year progression-free survival of about 45%. For patients with ALL beyond the first remission and subjected to an allogeneic SCT, following salvage chemotherapy, current results show a 5-year progression-free survival of about 30%. There has been little enthusiasm with regard to reduced-intensity SCT in ALL, largely because at present there is little evidence supporting the notion of a GvL effect in ALL.

Autologous transplantation for ALL

The role of autologous SCT remains unclear, despite encouraging preliminary results, with most comparative studies showing no major survival difference compared with chemotherapy. A small Italian study has suggested a possible role of autologous SCT in patients who sustain an early CNS relapse, but in general at present it is probably best to offer this treatment only as part of a clinical trial.

Chronic myeloid leukemia (CML)

Allogeneic transplantation for CML

Allogeneic SCT using an HLA-matched donor, performed in the chronic phase (CP) of chronic myeloid leukemia (CML) can cure selected patients with CML and cure depends on the contribution of the GvL effect (see above). Registry collated data (CIBMTR) reveal the probability of progression-free survival at 5 years is 55–60%. The probability of relapse at 5 years was 15% (see Figures 9.7 and 9.8). In contrast the results of allogeneic SCT performed in more advance phases of the disease are generally poor. The major determinants for survival, other than the phase of the disease, include the patient's age at transplant, the CMV status of the patient, and the age and sex of the donor. Survival appears to be best for patients who are transplanted within 1 year of diagnosis, are less than 40 years of age, have a young male donor, and both patient and donor are CMV seronegative. For such a cohort, the 5-year progression-free survival is probably around 70–80% with a relapse rate of 10–20%. It is possible that the precise details of the transplant procedure and the choice of stem cells (bone marrow vs. peripheral blood) also influence the outcome. There has also been some concern with regard to the effect of prior IFN-α therapy following an initial observation suggesting a possible detrimental effect and further careful monitoring is warranted.

The best results from allogeneic SCT are from an HLA-identical sibling donor, though such a donor is only available for less than 30% of patients eligible for SCT. The results of matched unrelated donor (MUD) SCT were in the past inferior to those of sibling SCT due to the increased rate of graft failure, GvHD and transplant-related mortality, although recent results

185

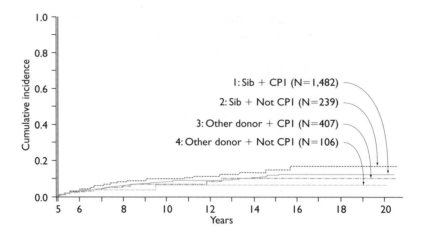

Figure 9.7   The probability of relapse at 5 years for patients with chronic myeloid leukemia who receive an HLA-matched sibling donor stem cell transplant [reproduced with permission from the CIBMTR report (2003)].

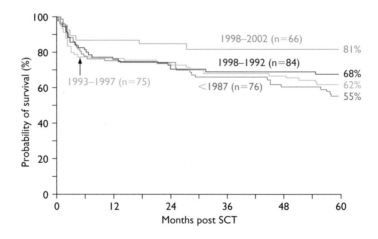

Figure 9.8   The probability of disease-free survival at 5 years for 301 patients with chronic myeloid leukemia who received an HLA-matched sibling donor stem cell transplant at the Hammersmith Hospital, London, UK [data collated in September 2003].

suggest that the disparity in survival rates have diminished greatly or indeed disappeared. The presence of GvHD greatly increases the risk of transplant-related problems following an allogeneic SCT from infections. Current results from the Seattle group suggest a progression-free survival of 57% at 5 years in patients who were under the age of 55 years and a progression-free survival of 74% for patients under the age of 50 years who were transplanted within 1 year of diagnosis. Clearly these results are remarkable and approach the cure rates accorded by HLA-matched sibling donors. Syngeneic SCT in CML has a comparable overall survival to sibling SCT, but owing to the lack of a GvL effect there is a higher relapse rate resulting in a lower progression-free survival. Allogeneic SCT from other family members who are partially matched requires intensive conditioning regimens and has a higher toxicity from GvHD and graft failure.

Specialists have been assessing the potential role of reduced-intensity allogeneic SCT for patients with CML with great optimism in view of the GvL effect which is probably maximal in this disease. It is possible to achieve full donor chimerism (see above) and eradication of cytogenetic and molecular evidence of CML is sometimes achieved. Patients who are partial chimeras can be converted to full chimeras with DLI. Recent experiences suggest a progression-free survival at 5 years of about 85% (see Figure 9.9). There is also some enthusiasm to explore the use of a reduced-intensity SCT for patients with CML, following a cytogenetic remission with imatinib. Conversely reduced-intensity SCT could be used in newly diagnosed patients followed by imatinib.

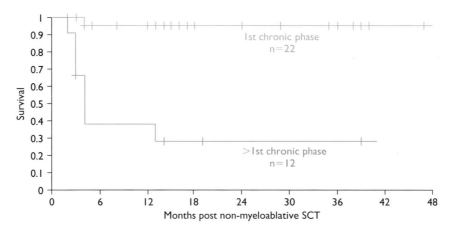

Figure 9.9   The probability of disease-free survival at 5 years for 34 patients with chronic myeloid leukemia (sibling SCT=22; unrelated SCT=12) who received a reduced-intensity stem cell transplant [reproduced with permission from Or *et al.* (2003) Nonmyeloablative allogeneic stem cell transplantation for the treatment of chronic myeloid leukemia in first chronic phase, *Blood* 101: 441–5].

Treatment for relapse of CML post-allogeneic transplant

In the 10–20% of patients who relapse post-allogeneic SCT for CML, this occurs in the first 3 years. This relapse tends to follow an orderly progression with the patient initially demonstrating evidence of a molecular relapse, followed by a cytogenetic relapse when the Ph chromosome is found, and then hematological and clinical relapse. Molecular monitoring of all SCT recipients is therefore valuable. For patients with molecular relapse, remission can be re-induced simply by withdrawal of immunosuppression or by the transfusion of donor lymphocytes (DLI). DLI can induce remissions in 60–80% of patients with molecular or cytogenetic relapse. Patients who fail to enter remission with DLI may be treated with imatinib mesylate (see Chapter 8). They may also be candidates for a second allogeneic SCT but the risk of transplant-related problems, including death, is relatively high.

Autologous transplantation for CML

Autologous SCT following high-dose chemotherapy can prolong survival for patients with CML. It is now also widely recognized that some Ph-negative stem cells survive at the time of diagnosis in most patients, lending support to efforts being made to develop autografting techniques that favor reconstitution with Ph-negative hemopoiesis (presumably normal hemopoiesis). Some studies suggest that this can indeed be achieved in a minority of patients and is durable in some cases. For the most part, autologous SCT for CML is reserved as part of clinical trials.

How to make transplant treatment decisions for individual patients with CML in 2005?

Since the successful introduction of imatinib (Glivec; Gleevec) into the clinic for patients with CML, the role of allogeneic SCT, the only treatment known to result in a long-term molecular remission and likely cure, posed a quandary, both for the patient and the specialist. Current experience with imatinib suggests that though the vast majority of patients achieve a hematological remission, very few enter a molecular remission and therefore probably are not cured. *Pari passu* there has been a significant advance in the increasing availability of allogeneic SCT through reduced-intensity allogeneic SCT. This latter advance makes it difficult to rely on the currently validated prognostic scores, which were designed to help decide a treatment strategy commensurate with the individual's disease-related (Euro score) and transplant-related (Gratwohl score) risks. Gratwohl's score is based on five well-defined prognostic factors for survival following a conventional allo-SCT: donor type (matched sibling vs. unrelated), recipient's age, the stage of the disease, the sex of the donor and recipient, and the interval from diagnosis to allo-SCT (Figure 9.10). It is likely that, in future, genomic testing will provide significant prognostic information, which will be helpful in selecting the appropriate therapy for an individual patient (Figure 9.11).

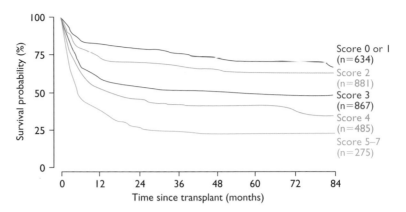

Figure 9.10   European Blood and Marrow Transplant (EBMT) Group's scoring system for patients with chronic myeloid leukemia in chronic phase being considered for an allogeneic stem cell transplant. [adapted, with permission, from Gratwohl et al 1998, *Lancet*, Oct 2].

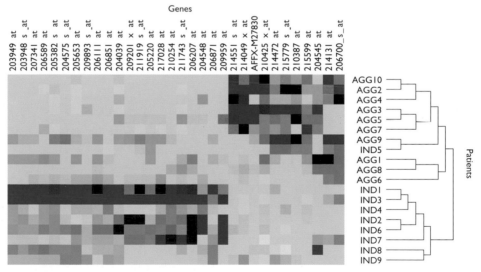

Figure 9.11   DNA microarray analysis of a cohort of patients with CML in chronic phase [adapted, with permission from Yong et al, 2005 Blood on-line September 2005].

Currently we feel that one may consider initial treatment by allogeneic SCT for any young patient with an optimal donor and wishes to be transplanted, but unquestionably the great majority of patients should start treatment with

189

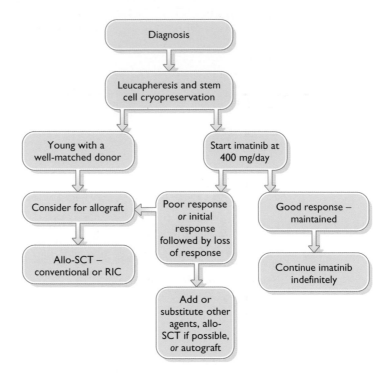

Figure 9.12   Suggested algorithm for the treatment of chronic myeloid leukemia [reproduced with permission from Goldman and Mughal (2005) Chronic myeloid leukemia. *Postgraduate Hematology*, eds Hoffbrand and Catovsky, Blackwell Science, Oxford, UK].

imatinib. Patients with possible transplant donors who fail imatinib should be considered for an allogeneic SCT (Figure 9.12).

Stem cell transplantation for chronic lymphocytic leukemia (CLL)

Preliminary results with allogeneic and autologous SCT for the treatment of advanced-stage chronic lymphocytic leukemia (CLL) in young adults demonstrate high- and long-lasting response rates, including molecular remissions, suggesting that this treatment may offer the chance of cure to selected patients with poor-risk CLL. Recent results collated by the registries (EBMT and CIBMTR) confirm the applicability of SCT, both allogeneic and autologous, for the treatment of patients with Rai/Binet poor-risk CLL who are under the age of 50 years. The 5-year progression-free survival for the patients who received an allogeneic SCT was 34% and for those who received an autologous SCT it was 28%; the risk of relapse was 40% and 70%, respectively. These preliminary experiences are encouraging and further studies are in progress. The potential role of reduced-intensity allogeneic SCT is also being assessed.

Myelodysplastic syndrome (MDS)

Allogeneic transplantation for MDS

Allogeneic SCT, using an HLA-matched sibling donor, offers the only chance of achieving a cure to a small proportion of patients with myelodysplastic syndrome (MDS). Historically the results of allogeneic transplant in these patients have been considerably poorer than those with AML without MDS owing to a higher relapse rate. It has been speculated that the higher disease burden and poor prognosis cytogenetic features present in many of the MDS patients may be the major factors. There is, however, some uncertainty with regard to the use of chemotherapy prior to SCT and the importance of the disease burden. Current results of allogeneic SCT using HLA-matched sibling donors and more effective conditioning regimens have led to better results, with a long-term progression-free survival of about 75% for patients under the age of 40 years. Results of allogeneic SCT using matched unrelated donors have also improved with transplantation earlier in the course of the disease and better conditioning and recent results show a progression-free survival of about 39% after 3 years of follow-up.

It is possible that further progress may result from the use of non-myeloablative allogeneic SCT followed by donor lymphocyte infusions. Such an approach should be particularly suitable for the older patients. In September 2004, Ghulam Mufti and colleagues in London reported early results on 62 patients with MDS, aged 41–70 years, who received non-myeloablative allogeneic SCT (24 patients had HLA-matched sibling donors and 38 had matched unrelated donors) following conditioning with fludarabine, busulfan and Campath 1-H (alemtuzumab). The overall survival at 1 year was 73% for siblings and 71% for unrelated donors, with a progression-free survival of 61% and 59%, respectively (Figure 9.13). Clearly these results are quite promising and longer follow-up is required.

Autologous transplantation for MDS

Autologous SCT may be useful for patients who achieve a remission following chemotherapy and are not suitable for an allogeneic SCT. This concept gains support from the observation that some patients with MDS exhibit normal hemopoiesis following chemotherapy. Current studies assessing the value of autologous SCT following chemotherapy in patients with high-risk MDS suggest progression-free survival of about 30% at 2 years, though the relapse rates were high.

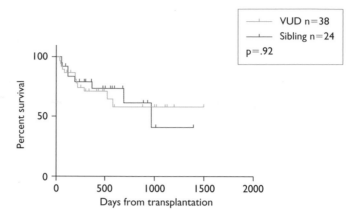

Figure 9.13   The probability of disease-free survival at 1 year for patients with myelodysplastic syndrome who receive a reduced-intensity stem cell transplant [reproduced with permission from Ho *et al.* (2004) Reduced-intensity allogeneic hemopoietic stem cell transplantation for myelodysplastic syndrome and acute myeloid leukemia with multilineage dysplasia using fludarabine, busulphan, and alemtuzumab (FBC) conditioning, *Blood* 104: 1616–23].

Lymphomas

Stem cell transplantation for non-Hodgkin lymphomas

Patients with high-grade lymphomas, who present with multiple adverse risk factors, should be offered an autologous SCT as soon as they achieve a first remission with chemotherapy. Current experience suggests that as many as 55% of these patients can achieve a long-term remission and possible cure with such an approach (Figure 9.14). The overall 5-year survival of such patients is also increased to about 75%, compared with 45% after CHOP (Figure 9.15). Autologous SCT is also the most effective form of therapy for patients who relapse following chemotherapy for high-grade lymphoma. Many specialists offer such patients a brief course of chemotherapy to reduce the disease bulk prior to proceeding with the transplant. Patients who progress during the initial chemotherapy (refractory disease) or who fail to respond to the initial doses of the salvage chemotherapy (resistant disease) have a significantly lower chance of responding to the autologous SCT.

Patients with low-grade lymphomas, such as follicular lymphoma, will ultimately fail whatever conventional therapy they have been offered. Both autologous and allogeneic SCT have been shown to produce long-term disease-free survival in a proportion of such patients. Allogeneic SCT is associated with a higher mortality rate, but there is reasonably convincing evidence

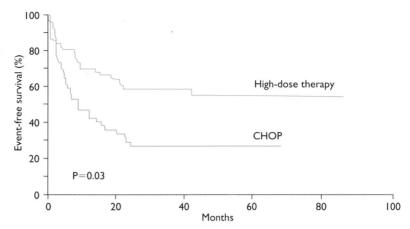

Figure 9.14   The probability of disease-free survival at 5 years for patients with lymphomas who receive an autologous stem cell transplant [reproduced with permission from Milpied *et al.* (2004) Initial treatment of aggressive lymphoma with high dose chemotherapy and autologous stem-cell support, *N Engl J Med* 350: 1287–95].

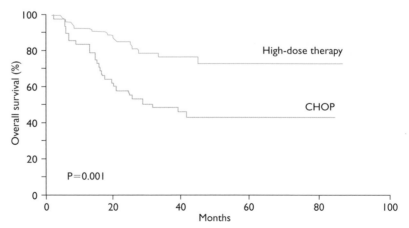

Figure 9.15   The probability of disease-free survival at 5 years for patients with lymphomas treated with an autologous stem cell transplant as part of the first-line treatment compared with conventional CHOP treatment alone [reproduced with permission from Milpied *et al.* (2004) Initial treatment of aggressive lymphoma with high dose chemotherapy and autologous stem-cell support, *N Engl J Med* 350: 1287–95].

available for its potential to produce a cure in some of these patients, probably as a result of a graft-versus-lymphoma effect. It has been observed that even patients who had previously received multiple treatments can achieve remissions with an allogeneic SCT. This has paved the way to many efforts being directed to offer a reduced-intensity SCT to patients with lymphoma.

Stem cell transplantation for Hodgkin lymphoma

About 30% of patients treated with chemotherapy for advanced stages of Hodgkin lymphoma, sadly, will suffer relapse after achieving a remission. Those who relapse within a year of completing therapy or never achieve a first remission have a poor prognosis. Autologous SCT has proven to allow up to 50% of such patients to enter a long-lasting remission and possible cure.

Patients who relapse after achieving a continuous remission for over 2 months can usually enter a second remission with chemotherapy. However, the majority of these patients do relapse again and many specialists recommend an autologous SCT for them.

Myelomas

Autologous stem cell transplantation for myeloma

Autologous SCT for patients with myeloma are now almost exclusively performed with peripheral blood stem cells since the cells engraft rapidly and are less likely to be contaminated with myeloma cells, in contrast to bone marrow-derived cells. Current results suggest that the progression-free survival is increased by about 12 months with intensive therapy and autologous SCT compared with standard chemotherapy (Figure 9.16). Patients with the poorest prognosis appear to obtain a greater survival benefit with the intensive treatment.

Some centers offer 'tandem' autologous transplants (two autologous transplants carried out in sequence) as a mean of attempting to deliver more effective eradication of disease. A recent French randomized study, however, failed to show a major difference between the single versus double autologous transplants, and most specialists only offer a tandem transplant in a clinical trial setting.

It is important to realize that an autologous SCT will not cure the majority of patients, but rather reduces the burden of myeloma cells to a level where many patients achieve a status approaching an 'operational cure' (whereby the patient has persistent molecular disease, but is free of any major stigmas of the disease and does not require any specific therapy, see Chapter 8), since they do not have any of the major consequences of myeloma and might not

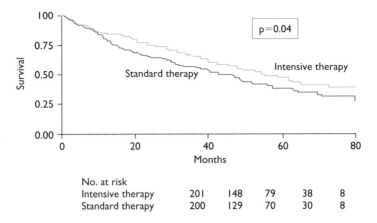

Figure 9.16   The probability of disease-free survival at 5 years for patients with myeloma who receive an autologous stem cell transplant [reproduced with permission from Childs *et al.* (2003) High-dose chemotherapy with hemopoietic stem-cell rescue for multiple myeloma, *N Engl J Med* 348: 1875–83].

even require any specific anti-myeloma therapy. For these reasons, there is considerable enthusiasm in assessing the possibility of following an autologous transplant, either single or tandem, with a reduced-intensity allogeneic transplant, as discussed above. There are also a number of other novel trials, such as the use of thalidomide, bortezomib (Velcade) and vaccine therapy following an autologous transplant to convert the low-volume disease (typically slightly more than what is considered 'minimal residual disease') to a complete cure. Efforts are also being directed to 'purge' the harvested stem cells of residual myeloma cells, to minimize contamination, which can lead to relapse.

Most specialists will offer induction chemotherapy, often the VAD combination (see Chapter 8), to reduce the myeloma burden, following which the patients can be subjected to an autologous SCT. Patients who do not fare well with the chemotherapy usually tend to fare less well with the transplant, though rarely, some patients go on to achieve an excellent result with a transplant for their chemotherapy-resistant disease. Some specialists may offer induction therapy with thalidomide, with or without dexamethasone.

Allogeneic stem cell transplantation for myeloma

Allogeneic SCT appears to offer a 35% chance of long-term progression-free survival and possible cure, but the transplant-related mortality is excessively high at about 25%, probably due to GvHD, lung inflammations and relapse. Despite these difficulties, it remains the only form of currently available

195

treatment which offers the chance of a molecular remission and a possible cure, largely as a result of the GvM effect. For this reason, many specialists continue to consider younger patients (age less than 55 years) who have an HLA-matched sibling donor and wish to be transplanted, for this procedure. This effect is now being exploited by offering patients a reduced-intensity allogeneic SCT, which should lower the high transplant-related mortality. Patients who respond to this poorly or relapse thereafter can be treated with donor lymphocyte infusions (DLI), with or without thalidomide. The role of reduced-intensity SCT is also being assessed following an autologous SCT, a modification of the conventional 'tandem' transplants.

Stem cell transplantation for systemic amyloidosis

The prognosis of systemic amyloidosis (AL disease) is in general quite poor, but hematological complete remissions, improvement of target organ dysfunction, and improved overall survival have been reported following SCT, in particular allogeneic for those who are eligible for this procedure. Most patients, however, are not eligible, and should be considered for an autologous SCT, though the transplant-related mortality is high for those with cardiac involvement.

10 *Side-effects of the treatment of leukemias, lymphomas and myelomas*

The advances in the treatment of leukemias, lymphomas and myelomas have allowed many patients to achieve long-lasting remissions, and perhaps, cure. Consequently more and more people are looking at the quality of life after treatment. Cancer therapy can be associated with both acute and delayed detrimental effects. Much attention has, therefore, focused on the consequences of such effects on patients. Such efforts show that although most side-effects, particularly the acute effects, are largely preventable and many supportive measures can make the cancer therapy more tolerable, a significant minority of long-term cancer survivors face socio-economic and medical problems of a diverse nature, particularly children and young adults. For example, children who were subjected to radiation treatment to the central nervous system as part of their leukemia treatment plan and appeared to have been cured of leukemia were found to have death rates much higher than expected. These children were also noted to face much higher levels of unemployment compared with those children who did not receive radiation. As cancer specialists, we have an enormous responsibility to all survivors to continue to be vigilant and anticipate and identify problems that patients may encounter after therapy and help them lead lives that are as normal and productive as possible.

Generally speaking, chemotherapy used for the treatment of blood cancers can cause a number of acute or short-term effects which are transient and fully reversible. Such effects include severe nausea and vomiting, hair loss, fatigue, infections related to treatment-induced low white blood cell counts and may have implications for fertility. The delayed side-effects are very rare but significant since they can sometimes result in a higher mortality rate than the disease itself and can be a major problem for the patients who appear to have been cured of their disease. Radiotherapy effects depend on the site (area) being treated but tend to be more localized, but delayed effects include secondary cancers.

Acute side-effects

Nausea and vomiting

Nausea and vomiting induced by cancer therapy in general are probably the most bothersome short-term effects. The incidence and severity of nausea and vomiting in the treatment of blood cancers with combination chemotherapy is quite high, involving about 70 to 75% of all patients receiving such therapy. Anticipatory nausea and vomiting, which commences about a day before the patient actually starts anti-cancer therapy, is experienced by about a third of the patients and can become a problem as the treatment cycles proceed. In the majority of patients good control can be achieved by the use of the modern anti-emetic agents such as ondansetron (Zofran), granisetron (Kytril), aprepitant (Emend), palonosetron (Aloxi) and dolasetron (Anzemet) in conjunction with steroids such as dexamethasone; anticipatory nausea and vomiting is helped considerably by prescribing drugs such as lorazepam (Ativan), which relaxes the patients and can be commenced about 12 hours ahead of the treatment.

Oral complications

Oral (mouth) problems that develop during the course of cancer therapy are often related to diverse factors. Mucositis is a term often used by specialists and others to describe oral symptoms a patient may experience (Figure 10.1). Oral mucositis can be defined as an inflammation of the mucous membrane of the oral cavity. It is a significant problem for almost all cancer patients receiving therapy because of immunosuppression and the cytotoxic effect on a rapid turnover of oral mucosa. Its prevalence in non-transplant patients seems to be about 40%, rising to almost 80% for those undergoing high-dose therapy and stem cell transplantation. Regular mouth care and the use of mouth washes can help preventing it. For patients with established mucositis, a number of remedies such as sucralfate and nystatin mouth washes can help; capsaicin, the active ingredient in chili pepper may also be useful, particularly in alleviating mucositis-associated pain. Oral infections, such as candida (yeast), are a particular problem and can be treated with fluconazole.

(a) (b)

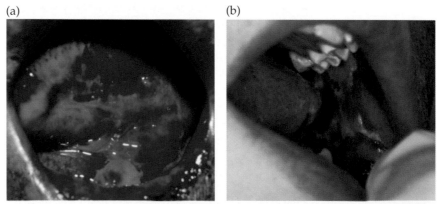

Figure 10.1   (a) Severe ulceration and obliteration of the muscle under the tongue in a patient receiving high-dose chemoradiotherapy and (b) ulceration of the cheek in a patient receiving high-dose chemotherapy (courtesy of Amgen Europe, Luzern, Switzerland).

Clinical trials are currently assessing the potential role of novel therapies such as keratinocytic growth factor (palifermin) and glutamine, which is an essential amino acid that regulates protein breakdown, prevents gut atrophy and enhances immune function.

Palifermin works by protecting the cells that line the mouth and gut from the damage caused by chemoradiotherapy. Current studies in patients receiving high-dose chemoradiotherapy and SCT have confirmed its efficacy and safety and led to its approval by US and European regulatory agencies.

Hair loss (alopecia)

Alopecia, in particular scalp hair loss, is a distressing, both physically and psychologically, and common side-effect of many of the drugs used to treat patients with blood cancers. It induces body image and interpersonal problems, which often begin soon after cancer therapy is commenced. In some cases the scalp hair loss is almost total, but fully reversible. The new hair is often curlier and might be of a lighter shade. Some institutions offer methods of scalp cooling, which may prevent hair loss in some patients by preventing the drugs from entering the scalp (and so pose a theoretical risk of residual cancer cells in the scalp blood vessels). Most patients prefer to cover their heads, either with scarves, turbans, hats or wigs. It is best for patients to select their preferred head covering before hair loss begins.

Bone marrow suppression

Chemotherapy-associated effects on the bone marrow are a potentially serious side-effect (see Chapter 8). For most of the drugs, the nadir is at 7 to 10 days, when patients will be at risk of acquiring an infection as a result of neutropenia. Specialists may prescribe prophylactic antibiotics, such as ciprofloxacin to cover the period of neutropenia and in some cases use G-CSFs to promote recovery of the neutrophils. Chemotherapy-associated anemia is common and may need to be treated promptly.

Markedly low platelet counts (thrombocytopenia) can also occur and may require the administration of platelet transfusions. Efforts are being directed to develop platelet-stimulating growth factor therapy, such as interleukin-11 or thrombopoietin (Neumega; oprelvekin).

Nerve damage (neuropathy)

This can be seen in patients receiving drugs, such as the vinca alkaloids, for example vincristine and vinblastine, and thalidomide bortezomib. Typically the patient complains of pins and needles or tingling sensation in hands, feet or both. Rarely it results in jaw pain and paralysis of the small bowel (ileum). In most cases, the neuropathy is mild and improves over weeks to months, on reducing or even discontinuing the suspected drug. In rare cases it may pose a long-term problem and drugs such as neurontin and pyridoxine may help some patients.

Kidney problems (nephropathy)

The kidneys are often the most pertinent organs for eliminating drugs and their metabolites (products of the drugs as they are destroyed by the body), and can therefore be vulnerable. Drugs, such as methotrexate, are typically involved and patients may develop abnormal biochemical kidney tests, with no major clinical consequences, or which can result in significant kidney problems requiring dialysis. The specialists will be wary and undertake steps to safeguard the kidneys when using drugs which pose such a risk.

Liver problems (hepatotoxicity)

Many of the drugs used can cause liver problems, typically mild and not significant enough to result in any clinical sequel. They can cause chemical hepatitis and liver cellular dysfunction which can result in an alteration of liver enzymes (biochemistry) and lead to problems with some other drugs, such as blood 'thinners' like warfarin (Coumadin), which the patient may be taking for an unrelated disease. Drugs used in the treatment of ALL, such as L-asparaginase, appear to have a high incidence of liver toxicity. Rarely the treatment can result in changes in the venous outflow from liver cells and result in 'veno-occlusive' liver disease. This is seen with cytarabine, cyclophosphamide and in the combinations used for conditioning treatments in the stem cell transplantation setting. Some drugs, such methotrexate, can result in 'fibrosis' if used for long periods.

Heart problems (cardiotoxicity)

Some drugs, such as the anthracyclines (see Chapter 8), can cause damage to the heart muscle, which is usually related to high doses, but rarely can occur at low doses. It results in dilatation of the heart chambers and is usually irreversible. Specialists will therefore try their best to minimize this from arising by monitoring the doses, assessing the cardiac function periodically and assessing the role of cardio-protective agents in clinical trials.

Bone problems (necrosis)

Patients receiving steroids, particularly in high doses for long periods, as is often the case in particular in patients with ALL, are at risk of developing necrosis (aseptic) of the femoral heads (Figure 10.2). This is irreversible and requires most patients to discontinue the drug; surgical correction may be indicated.

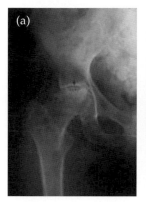
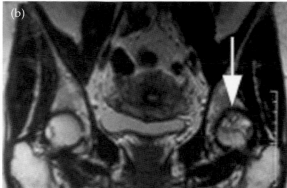

Figure 10.2   (a) An xray and (b) a MRI scan of the hip showing bone necrosis of the femoral heads in a patient on long-term steroid therapy.

Psychological issues

Sadly, as we mentioned earlier, the diagnosis of a cancer is still equated with a sense of hopelessness, fear and early (premature) death even today. The diagnosis and treatment produce a number of important psychological issues, both acute and delayed, which we are not able to discuss in great detail in a book like ours (see 'suggested reading', Appendix II). These issues encompass the normal psychological responses to cancer and its therapy; psychotropic effects of some of the chemotherapy drugs, and related topics such as the role of unconventional cancer therapies, sexual, cultural and spiritual counseling, and survivor issues. Cancer therapy is associated with significant disruptions in family, vocational, peer, school and employment domains. Paradoxically major stress can be associated with successful outcomes for cancer therapies also. Many patients can struggle with issues associated with resumption of family and other relationships, as well as social, leisure and employment issues and should be offered appropriate professional help. There are a number of community resources (see Appendix I), such as peer-support groups, which now form a crucial part of the cancer management team. The patient's closest contacts, both family and friends, clearly play an important role, particularly as a source of emotional support at all stages of the management, from diagnosis to therapy and beyond.

Late side-effects

Infertility

Infertility is particularly likely when young adults are subjected to an alkylating agent, such as chlorambucil or cyclophosphamide. The risk of infertility appears to be age related in women, but not men; women over the age of 30 years are particularly vulnerable. Fortunately, the majority of patients who have had chemotherapy, even aggressive chemotherapy, and stem cell transplantation or radiotherapy are able to conceive naturally and have perfectly healthy children. It is important for all patients of child-bearing age to be counseled on their fertility prospects prior to the initiation of anti-cancer therapy.

All patients of child-bearing age should receive advice about the effects of their planned treatment on fertility; the treatment rarely affects the actual ability to have intercourse, though libido is often decreased. It is often devastating for a young patient who may not have had any children to be told that he/she might not be able to do so as a direct result of the treatment. Generally the very young patients may not sustain much damage to the ovaries or testes, but it typically depends on the type and dose of drugs used. Many of the current drugs and the various combinations used today are less likely to result in reduction in fertility. In patients subjected to radiotherapy, it is possible (and mandatory) to shield the gonads (ovaries and testes) during exposure to radiotherapy and the lowest effective doses of radiation are used.

Men with some form of malignancy may have impaired fertility even before any specific treatment is commenced. This is often because the making of sperm by the testes (a process known as spermatogenesis) is easily affected by many types of illnesses. These observations have been based on many male patients who are referred for sperm banking, a procedure where sperms are collected, frozen (cryopreserved) and then stored (for up to 50 or more years!). It is likely that stress plays a large part, since these individuals would have had to deal with the diagnosis of a cancer and the potential treatment just days or weeks prior and then are requested to produce a sperm sample (semen) on demand.

Some specialists are exploring the possibility of freezing testicular tissue, obtained by biopsy. A single sperm is then isolated and injected into an egg (oocyte), which is then implanted into the uterus. This is known as *in vitro* fertilization (IVF) ('test-tube' baby treatment). The options available to women are to freeze eggs (oocytes), embryos or ovarian tissue. The freezing of oocytes is available at very few centers, which must be regulated by government agencies, and is often quite cumbersome with a small chance of a successful pregnancy at the end. Women need to go through a full ovarian stimulation procedure, the objective of which is to encourage the ovaries to produce mature oocytes, followed by a key-hole laparotomy (laparoscopy) whereby a hole is made in the abdomen and the oocytes (usually about 10) are collected and frozen. The technique has been used for over a decade, but so far very few successful pregnancies have been reported.

Embryo freezing, in contrast, is well recognized and has been offered for almost three decades. This also requires full ovarian stimulation followed by the laparoscopic removal of an oocyte, which is then fertilized *in vitro* with a sperm from the partner and the resulting embryo is then frozen. In due course, when the patient is ready to have a baby, the embryo is thawed and implanted into the uterus. This option, though not always successful, is probably the best current fertility treatment for women.

Ovarian tissue freezing is an experimental technique which has now been in an exploratory state for just under a decade. It requires the patient to undergo a laparoscopy to remove a small piece of one of the ovaries, before anti-cancer treatment is started. The piece of ovary is then frozen and stored in a specialist fertility unit. The objective here is to be able to transfer this piece back into the ovary or another site in the patient in the hope that it will 're-grow' and the ovarian tissue be able to produce normal oocytes in the future. It is also possible that a specialist might be able to isolate the immature oocytes from the tissue removed and culture them in order to obtain mature oocytes, which can then be fertilized by the partner's sperm and the result-ing embryo transferred back into the uterus. This technique can only be offered as part of a clinical trial.

Specialists may also discuss the role of donor sperm or donor eggs. Most patients will probably appreciate hearing this and will be reassured that even if their ovarian or testicular function remains poor, they can still become par-ents if they consider the use of donated sperm or donated eggs. The entire matter is quite sensitive and most patients are best served by appropriate advice from the specialists, often in conjunction with a fertility expert, and counseling might be helpful.

Second cancers

Second (new) cancers are a rare complication of previous chemotherapy and radiotherapy. The risk of developing a second cancer following either therapy alone, in conventional doses, is very small, but undoubtedly very serious; the risk is increased when they are used in combination or in high doses, such as in SCT. Patients treated with drugs, particularly DNA-damaging agents such as alkylating agents, can sometimes develop second-ary myelodysplastic syndromes (MDS) and acute leukemia, which we discussed in detail in Chapter 7. It should be remembered that not all second cancers are therapy related; some may represent a chance occurrence or might result from host (patient) susceptibility factors such as an immuno-deficiency or a genetic predisposition. For these reasons, it is important to study patients with second cancers in detail, particularly at a molecular level, which might reveal the mechanisms underlying chemotherapy- and radiotherapy-induced cancers further.

The risk of radiotherapy-related second cancers begins at about 10 years, but can be seen earlier. In contrast to conventional chemotherapy, where most of the second cancers tend to be MDS and acute leukemias, there is an increase in the risk of second solid cancers following radiotherapy. Recently an increased risk of breast cancer has been documented in young females with Hodgkin lymphoma, who were subjected to radiotherapy, either alone or in combination with chemotherapy. This is particularly devastating, since the prognosis of these secondary cancers can be poor. Young women should therefore be offered regular mammography and breast examinations. Young adults should be urged to refrain from smoking cigarettes to reduce the risk of lung cancer. For many cancer therapies, the long-term effects on second cancers are not yet known. Furthermore, we are adding new therapies continuously, and their risks need to be assessed.

Second cancers related to high-dose therapy and stem cell transplantation (SCT) can occur more frequently than those related to conventional chemotherapy and radiotherapy, with an incidence of approximately 2%; but this could be slightly higher as the follow-up period increases further, as epidemiological studies suggest a continuous increase over time. This is similar to the incidence of solid tumors after combined chemotherapy–radiotherapy for Hodgkin lymphoma, where (sadly) even longer follow-up has failed to show a decline in the incidence of new cancers. In contrast, the incidence of MDS and acute leukemias related to conventional chemotherapy appears to fall after about 10 years of the therapy. Most of the second cancers related to SCT tend to be hematological cancers, particularly MDS and acute leukemias and lymphomas; solid tumors are also seen, particularly following allogeneic SCT. The overall risk of developing a second cancer appears to be the highest for recipients of an allogeneic SCT; in contrast the risk of secondary MDS is probably highest following an autologous SCT.

The precise reasons for these second cancers are unclear and probably multifactorial, with alterations in the immune function, viruses, high doses of chemotherapy and radiotherapy all playing a role; the excessive incidence of MDS following an autologous SCT is related to the high dose chemotherapy, myeloablative conditioning regimens. Current registry data (from the IBMTR) suggest a cumulative incidence of second solid cancers at 5, 10 and 15 years after SCT to be 0.7%, 2.2% and 6.7%, respectively; the precise cumulative incidence of hematological cancers is higher with MDS exceeding 10% following autologous SCT. The risk was 8.3 times higher among those patients who survived 10 or more years after transplantation as compared with the general population. The most common solid cancers observed were melanoma (skin cancer) and head and neck cancers, followed by brain tumors, thyroid cancers, breast cancers, bone cancers, liver cancers, bowel cancers and lung cancers. The leading cause of death for transplant recipients remains recurrence of primary disease and deaths from second solid cancers account for about 6% of all deaths following an allogeneic SCT.

Radiotherapy-related effects

Radiotherapy-related acute side-effects include nausea and vomiting, skin burns and tiredness (fatigue). These effects are all related to the size of the radiotherapy field, the dose per fraction and the site of radiotherapy. Patients receiving radiotherapy to the head and neck regions usually develop mucositis and dryness of the mouth, which results from the unavoidable radiotherapy effects on the salivary glands resulting in a reduced salivary flow.

Radiotherapy-related delayed side-effects usually appear after long follow-up. Some patients develop a unique electric-like shock sensation down the spine and sometimes into the legs when they bend (flex) their neck. This, known as Lhermitte's syndrome (also known as 'barber chair phenomenon'), described by Jacques Lhermitte in Paris in 1924, is often transient and requires no further investigations. Despite modern radiotherapy techniques limiting heart and lung damage, some patients do develop lung (pulmonary) fibrosis and coronary artery disease. Patients who have had neck radiotherapy are at risk for hypothyroidism (low thyroid hormone), which can make them become sluggish and gain weight and should be monitored by blood tests. The most sinister delayed problem related to radiotherapy is the occurrence of a second cancer, which we discussed above.

11 *Future prospects*

We now live firmly in the 'genomic' era. The enormous advances witnessed in molecular biology of cancer, such as the understanding of specific molecular abnormalities and the application of this knowledge in providing an effective cancer treatment, will continue at an ever-quickening pace. As specialists in hematologic cancers, we have been fortunate to have acquired so much molecular knowledge over such a short period of time. Such knowledge has paved the way for effective targeted therapy, best exemplified by imatinib for chronic myeloid leukemia, and ATRA in acute promyelocytic leukemia.

Conventional cytotoxic chemotherapy has been a qualified success in the treatment of specific hematological cancers over the past three decades; it has produced long-term survival and probable cure for patients with childhood leukemias, Hodgkin lymphoma and subgroups of non-Hodgkin lymphomas and other leukemias, but at the cost of considerable toxicity for the patient. The advent of targeted therapy now complements and will eventually displace the use of classical cytotoxic drugs. It makes therapy well worth the risk of side-effects and the financial costs.

Recent studies have enabled us to define molecular subtypes of the different hematologic cancers, even those which are similar morphologically, and this should enable us to tailor specific therapies for specific molecular 'signatures'. We also understand the role of the bone marrow milieu (microenvironment) much better, particularly in regard to the various interactions which take place in the pathogenesis of the different hematologic cancers. We are beginning to understand the interactions between the tumor cells and the cellular microenvironment and how the aggressiveness of diseases like follicular lymphoma is mainly determined by the cellular microenvironment, rather than the lymphoma cells themselves.

This dominant effect of the microenvironment on the prognosis of a cancer probably reflects the importance of the immune cells in the biology and pathogenesis of hematologic cancers. Such observations lend support to the notion that the growth of some hematologic cancers is not always autonomous. A good example is the gastric MALT lymphomas associated with infection by the *Helicobacter pylori* bacterium; many patients with this lymphoma can be cured in their early stages by use of antibiotics that eradicate the infection. In some patients with B-CLL, there is evidence suggesting activation by antigens, which probably play a decisive role in the pathogenesis in these patients. If the critical components of the microenvironment in B-CLL or follicular lymphoma can be identified, we can anticipate new treatment options.

Unraveling the human genome has provided the framework for identification and validation of novel targeted therapies to improve patient outcome. In the future, gene microarray profiling will enable patient-specific selection of targeted therapies and will also provide the framework for development of more potent and less-toxic targeted therapies. We are very much aware that society expects much of us; for example in a joint press conference that marked the official completion of the human genome mapping project in June 2000, Bill Clinton and Tony Blair speculated that 'it is now conceivable that our children's children will know the term cancer only as a constellation of stars'. At the November 2004 conference when world experts involved in the genome project met in New York, Bill Clinton remained just as enthusiastic; Mike Dexter of the Wellcome Trust (London) stated that he ranked the project as more important 'than the invention of the wheel'. We feel that many of the objectives will take time to realize but sooner or later we will arrive at 'personalized' treatment for individual cancers.

We have had reasonable success in treating leukemias, lymphomas and myelomas; in some cases, particularly childhood leukemias, almost 80% of children achieve a long-term freedom from disease and probably cure. Despite these successes, however, much work remains. The treatment remains difficult and fairly toxic, particularly in patients with acute leukemias, many of whom are probably overtreated and so unnecessarily exposed to the risk of side-effects, in particularly the long term effects. It is therefore critical to identify additional prognostic variables that can be used to tailor therapy more precisely (tiptoeing along the efficacy–toxicity tightrope); we need also to discover new drugs which are safer and more effective in killing cancer cells but less likely to damage normal cells.

Classical cytotoxic chemotherapy drugs are generally non-specific in their capacity to kill cells such that rapidly growing hematological cancer cells are not distinguished from rapidly growing normal cells, notably those in the bone marrow, skin, hair and the gut. Molecularly targeted drugs, in contrast, work at specific key points in the cancer cell's pathway and allows for the distinction between cancer cells and normal cells (to a certain degree). The availability of more drugs which can be administered by mouth also makes cancer treatment convenient and less disruptive to lifestyle. Supportive care is improving and helps deal with treatment-related complications promptly and efficiently. Better supportive treatments, such as hemopoietic growth factors, make the delivery of specific anti-cancer treatments easier and safer.

Stem cell transplantation, both allogeneic and autologous, is well established in the treatment of hematological cancers, although it is surrounded by some controversies and remains a potentially highly toxic procedure. The past decade has produced significant changes. First, we now have new ideas as to how an allogeneic transplant actually works and this has resulted in the increasing use of reduced-intensity preparatory regimens, which are much less toxic and rely more on the still poorly understood phenomenon described as the graft-versus-tumor (GvT) effect.

The donor stem cells are an adjunct to chemotherapy, both through the additional cytotoxicity and the biological modification through the GvT effect. This has made transplantation more available than in the past, since some patients who would not have been considered as candidates for a conventional allogeneic transplant, either because of age or performance status, can today be offered a reduced-intensity transplant.

Second, we are increasingly using blood-derived hemopoietic stem cells which result in a faster engraftment than marrow-derived stem cells; their use may result in fewer relapses and improved survival. Furthermore in keeping with a general improvement in supportive care, transplant-related mortality and morbidity has continued to decline as management of infections, particularly those due to viruses and fungi, improves.

Major uncertainties remain as to the most appropriate timing as well as effectiveness of allogeneic transplantation. Randomized trials have proven very difficult to conduct, largely for logistic reasons, and much of the evidence stems from data (largely retrospective) collated by transplant registries, such as the CIBMTR and the EBMT, or historical controls. At the same time that the results of stem cell transplantation have improved, the results of chemotherapy have also become better. Moreover, the successful introduction of molecularly targeted therapies and other novel agents, such as angiogenesis inhibitors, have made non-transplant treatments effective and safer.

In the treatment of chronic myeloid leukemia, where transplantation is the only form of therapy resulting in a probable cure, it is of interest that the number of patients subjected to allogeneic transplantation declined significantly even before the first published results of treatment with imatinib. These clinical decisions often make matters more complicated since they are driven by anticipation (and excitement) rather than actual evidence (much like the stock market!). Current results show that imatinib does not usually induce molecular remissions and at present should not yet entirely replace allogeneic stem cell transplant for those patients who are suitable candidates; rather imatinib should be used in a manner which allows the best outcomes. The next few years should see emerging strategies, based on the results of clinical trials of current and newer therapies, which allow us to integrate allogeneic transplant and non-transplant treatments appropriately.

Autologous transplantation can be considered a form of rescue from increased cytotoxic chemotherapy since it does not provide the GvT effects accompanied by an allogeneic transplant. In an attempt to harness a potential GvT effect, many efforts are being made to induce specific immunotoxicity where there are tumor antigens that are amenable to immune suppression, in particular leukemias. A number of candidate leukemia-associated antigens, such as the Wilms tumor antigen, which is known to be overexpressed in a variety of myeloid leukemias and other cancers, have been identified and studies to assess the potential usefulness of such strategies are in progress. The use of autologous transplants continues to increase for patients with lymphomas, both Hodgkin and non-Hodgkin, myelomas and acute myeloid leukemias.

Both autologous and allogeneic stem cells also provide a method of isolating potential targets for gene therapy. Genetic engineering, which allows researchers to pluck genes from chromosomes, has facilitated gene therapy and allowed us to replace defective or missing genes or to add helpful genes for both acquired and inherited disorders. Gene therapy has been used successfully in treating children with severe combined immune deficiency (SCID) in which a key enzyme is missing owing to the lack of a specific gene. Currently many technical hurdles remain to be cleared before such therapy can be applied widely.

Cancer can be envisaged as a Darwinian struggle in which an early (progenitor) cell evolves or progresses over a series of 'life-span' hurdles. However, an alternative scenario, perhaps scientifically not so attractive, has been proposed by an eminent blood cancer scientist, Mel Greaves from the Leukemia Research Fund Centre, London. He suggests that 'evolution is a concept much easier to recognize than define or apply'. All things ultimately evolve: the puzzle is which one of a number of plausible or seemingly improbable pathways is taken.

In his recent book *Cancer: The Evolutionary Legacy* (see Appendix II) he illuminates the evolutionary trail. He argues that cancers are the ends of long, unbroken chains that extend back billions of years. He proposes that at both ends of a cancer lineage, single clones are selected by chance for survival, expansion, invasion and migration. In between is the harmony of life, where the behavior of individual cells is harnessed for the good of the person (as a whole). The chain that connects this past and the present is the DNA. DNA replication is inherently prone to error, and these errors provide 'fruit' for evolution (or progression). Selection acts as a filter that determines which mutations survive (or persist). The complete history of a cancer cell includes the making and breaking of the genetic controls needed for 'life'. Chance pervades the entire process because of the randomness of mutation, the ambiguities of selection and the rather blinded nature of evolution. Clearly lifestyle should alter the odds, shedding light on some of the well-studied environmental factors such as radiation and tobacco smoking. Inevitably, further studies of cancer should provide further information on the mysteries of evolution.

Finally we very much hope that through suitably orchestrated efforts, integrating our increasing knowledge of the different hematological cancers, coupled with the tremendous advances in imaging and laboratory-based technologies, we might be able to prevent or cure many cancers. The twenty-first century, so far, has been a period of tremendous growth in knowledge of the genomics of cancer medicine. This growth has laid the foundations for unprecedented progress which should result in the prevention or eradication of many of the hematological cancers, but there are also many challenges, particularly with regard to the financing of many of these advances, especially in the less-developed countries. In the wake of enormous optimism generated by recent trial results of the newer and 'more' novel targeted therapies, patients and healthcare providers are dismayed about the cost of these drugs. There is an increasing expectation to personalize approaches which will undoubtedly increase the efficacy of our treatments whilst decreasing its toxicity and, hopefully, costs.

Currently we find ourselves, sadly more and more, in the undesirable position of having to help some patients make decisions about whether the potential clinical benefits warrant the financial strains created, particularly if the patients are responsible for some, if not all of the financial bill. In one of the richest countries in the world, the US, this can cause major hardships, even when patients have only to make a 'small' payment towards their care. In the UK, with a largely socialized form of medicine, the government is not prepared to fund many of the new treatments until robust survival advantages have been established and verified by a government-funded regulatory agency, optimistically designated the National Institute for Clinical Excellence (NICE). This of course can take many years, and in the interim the patient must wait. Figure 11.1 probably summarizes these issues.

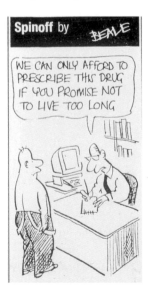

Figure 11.1   A cartoon epitomizing the increasing cost of today's drugs (courtesy of Mr Roger Beale)

Glossary

Acquired immune deficiency syndrome (AIDS)
A life-threatening disease caused by human immunodeficiency virus (HIV) and characterized by the breakdown of the body's immune system.

Acute (disease)
A disease described as acute is of short duration or rapid onset. The term does not imply severity.

Acute lymphoblastic leukemia (ALL)
A form of acute leukemia which affects the lymphoid cells. It is the most common form of childhood leukemia and also the most successfully treated.

Acute myeloid leukemia (AML)
The most common form of acute leukemia in adults.

Acute promyelocytic leukemia (APL)
A subtype of AML which often presents with abnormal bleeding/clotting and can often be successfully treated with AU-*trans*-retinoic acid (ATRA)

Acyclovir
An antiviral drug effective against herpes viruses; also know as Zovirax.

Adjunctive therapy
Treatment that is given either in preparation for or with definitive treatment. This should not be confused with adjuvant therapy which is treatment given after a complete surgical resection and all clinical evidence of a tumour removed; its purpose is to improve the long-term survival by killing molecular disease.

Adriamycin
A cytotoxic drug which is useful in the treatment of many forms of cancers, including leukemias, lymphomas and myelomas.

Adult T-cell leukemia/lymphoma (ATL)
A rare distinct form of chronic leukemia, causally associated with the HTLV-I infection.

Alemtuzumab
A monoclonal antibody treatment useful in the treatment of patients with chronic lymphocytic leukemia and in allogeneic stem cell transplantation; also known as Campath-1H.

Allele
Alternative forms (sequence) of a given gene.

Allogeneic stem cell transplant
A stem cell transplant between individuals other than identical twins.

Allopurinol
A drug which is effective in treating raised uric acid levels, which are sometimes found in patients with hematological cancers and gout; also useful in the treatment of tumour lysis syndrome (see below); also know as Zyloprim.

Aloxi
A drug which prevents or reduces nausea and vomiting related to chemotherapy; also known as palonosetron.

Ambisome
A lipid formulation of amphotericin B, with considerably fewer side-effects (see below).

Amphotericin B
A powerful anti-fungal drug.

Anaplastic lymphoma
A unique form of lymphoma which has an aggressive-looking appearance, but is probably one of the most curable forms.

Anemia
A decrease in the normal number of red blood cells and, therefore, the hemoglobin concentration of the blood. This results in a deceased ability of the blood to carry oxygen.

Angiogenesis
The development of new blood vessels within tumors. Therapies, such as thalidomide, that target them are called anti-angiogenesis.

Antibody
A protein molecule secreted by plasma cells (B lymphocytes) as a response to an antigen.

Antigen
A substance that is recognized by the body as foreign and capable of inducing an immune response.

Anti-thymocyte globulin
A drug which is often used to treat GvHD.

Anzemet
A drug that prevents or reduces nausea and vomiting related to chemotherapy; also known as dolasetron.

Apheresis
The selective removal of specific cells from a patient's body by means of a cell separator. When large numbers of white blood cells are removed, the process is referred to as leukapheresis; when platelets are removed, it is called plateletpheresis.

Apoptosis
A form of cell death which demonstrates the human body's ability to self-destruct (cell suicide).

Aprepitant
A drug which prevents or reduces nausea and vomiting related to chemotherapy; also known as Emend.

Aranesp
A long-acting erythropoietin molecule used in the treatment of anemia; the generic name is darbopoietin alfa.

Arsenic trioxide
A novel drug which is effective in acute promyelocytic leukemia, myelodysplastic syndromes and myelomas; also known as Trisenox.

Asparaginase
An anti-cancer drug given as part of the initial treatment of acute lymphoblastic leukemia.

ATRA
All-*trans*-retinoic acid, a vitamin A derivative useful in the treatment of acute promyelocytic leukemia.

Autologous stem cell transplant
A form of stem cell transplant where a patient's own stem cells are used. The technique is also referred to as autografting.

Azacytidine
A drug which can be effective in myelodysplastic syndrome; also known as 5-azacytidine (Vidaza).

B lymphocytes
Lymphocytes originating in the bone marrow.

Basophil
A type of leukocyte which plays an important role in a specific allergic reaction, known as an immediate hypersensitivity reaction.

Biological response modifiers
A diverse group of agents, often naturally occurring in humans, that can be produced by recombinant DNA technology and work by affecting the immune system.

Blast cell
Primitive blood cells appearing in large numbers in the bone marrow of patients with leukemias.

Blast crisis
The transition of chronic myeloid leukemia from an indolent chronic phase to an aggressive phase, resembling acute leukemias.

Bleomycin
A drug which is effective as part of combination chemotherapy for the treatment of Hodgkin lymphoma and other cancers.

Bone marrow transplant
See stem cell transplant.

Bortezomib
A new and effective treatment for myeloma; also known as Velcade.

Burkitt's lymphoma
A particular form of high-grade lymphoma; in Africa it is associated with the Epstein–Barr virus.

Busulfan
A drug which was a popular treatment for chronic myeloid leukemia in the 1970s and is now used as part of the conditioning treatments in stem cell transplants.

Cell cytoplasm
The contents of a cell, other than its nucleus.

Cell membrane
The other 'skin' of a cell.

Cell nucleus
The central organ of a cell that contains the information it needs to reproduce.

Cell immunity
The part of the immune system that protects the individual from infection by the actions of T lymphocytes.

Chimerism
The Chimera in mythology was a creature which had the head of a lion, the body of a goat and the tail of a serpent. In cancer medicine the term describes an organism whose body contains cell populations from different individuals of the same of different species occurring either spontaneously or created artificially.

Chlorambucil
A cytotoxic drug often used to treat chronic lymphocytic leukemia; also known as Leukeran.

Chromosomal translocation
An abnormality of chromosomes which occurs when a piece of one chromosome breaks off and sticks to the end of another chromosome. In a balanced translocation, a part of two chromosomes breaks off and the lost piece sticks to the broken end of the other chromosome.

Chromosome
'Strings' of DNA in the nuclei of cells consisting of genes.

Chronic lymphocytic leukemia (CLL)
The most common type of leukemia overall, mainly affecting older people.

Chronic myeloid leukemia (CML)
A rare form of leukemia with a well defined underlying molecular pathogenesis. This was the first human malignancy in which an effective milecularly targeted treatment was established.

Chronic myelomonocytic leukemia (CMML)
A chronic leukemia which has been included in the FAB categorization of myelodysplastic syndromes.

Cladribine
A drug which is effective in the treatment of hairy cell leukemia; also known as 2-chlorodeoxyadenosine (2CdA).

Clinical trials
Treatment protocols designed to seek and assess new treatments in a carefully controlled and ethical manner.

Clonal (monoclonal)
A population of cells derived from a single cell which may or may not be malignant.

Combination chemotherapy
Cytotoxic chemotherapy involving more than one drug; the drugs are usually combined to take advantage of their different modes of actions and potential synergism.

Complete remission
The disappearance of all known evidence of disease determined by two assessments not less than 4 weeks apart.

Computed tomography scan (CT)
X-ray computed tomography is a technique which provides non-invasive and cross-sectional body images. It was first introduced at the Atkinson Morley Hospital, London by Godfrey Hounsfield in 1972 (for which he was awarded the Nobel Prize in 1979). CT produces a series of cross-sectional images, usually in the axial plane (hence the acronym CAT scan, standing for computed axial tomography).

Conditioning treatment
Specialized treatment used for the preparation of the recipient for a stem cell transplant.

Consolidation treatment
Treatment given following a confirmed complete remission, aimed at killing any minimal quantities of disease left behind by the induction treatment.

Cord blood transplant
Use of umbilical cord blood-derived stem cells for allogeneic stem cell transplantation.

Cryopreservation
The freezing and subsequent storage of hemopoietic stem cells.

Cyclophosphamide
A powerful cancer drug used in the treatment of all the different kinds of hematological (and other) cancers; also known as Cytoxan.

Cyclosporine
A potent immunosuppressive drug used to treat GvHD; also known as cyclosporin A, Sandimmune or Neoral.

Cytarabine
A drug which is an effective treatment of leukemias; also known as cytosine arabinoside or Ara-C.

Cytogenetic remission
The disappearance of all known evidence of an abnormal karyotype (chromosome set) as determined by at least two evaluations by conventional or FISH (fluorescence *in situ* hybridization) techniques not less than 4 weeks apart.

Cytogenetics
The analysis of chromosomes in cells. It became possible as the result of a technique, known as chromosome banding, first introduced in 1969 by Torbjörn Caspersson and Lore Zech. The application of cytogenetics to hematological malignancies provides enormous information.

Cytokines
Biological molecules that the body produces in response to specific stimuli. They assist in the orderly operation of the body's defense responses and include such proteins as interferons and interleukins.

Cytomegalovirus
A herpes group virus that is particularly dangerous after allogeneic stem cell transplant.

Cytotoxic chemotherapy
Drugs which are used to kill cancer cells; also referred to as anti-cancer drugs.

Dacarbazine
A drug which is effective in the treatment of Hodgkin lymphoma; also known as DTIC.

Dasatinib
A novel drug which is useful in treating patients with imatinib-resistant chronic myeloid leukemia.

Daunorubicin
See adriamycin (above).

Dexamethasone
A steroid which is often used to prevent or reduce nausea and vomiting associated with chemotherapy. It is also used in the treatment of a number of hematological cancers, particular myelomas, and in cancers involving the central nervous system; also known as decadron.

Diffuse large B-cell lymphoma
The most common form of lymphoma, with an aggressive biological behavior which is quite responsive to chemotherapy; also known as large cell lymphoma.

Disseminated Intravascular Coagulation (DIC)
A bleeding/clotting condition which results from an inappropriate activation of the coagulation (clotting) system. It is often seen in patients with leukemia, particularly APL.

DNA
Deoxyribonucleic acid is the genetic material present in every cell.

Donor lymphocyte infusion (DLI)
A procedure with which it is often possible to convert patients with hematological cancers, in particular chronic myeloid leukemia, who show mixed chimerism (see above) following an allogeneic stem cell transplant, to a full donor chimera and therefore complete remission.

Doxil
A liposomal encapsulated form of the powerful drug, daunorubicin (adriamycin).

Emend
See aprepitant.

Engraftment
The process in which donor hematopoietic stem cells infused into the recipient migrate to the bone marrow and begin to grow and produce new blood cells.

Eosinophil
A type of leukocyte which plays an important role in the response to parasitic and allergic diseases.

Erythrocytes
Cells which are responsible for carrying oxygen and carbon dioxide to and from the lungs; also known as red blood cells.

Erythropoietin
A biological molecule (cytokine) which stimulates the production of red blood cells.

Etoposide
A drug used to treat some patients with hematological cancers; also known as VP16.

Extranodal
The presence of lymphatic tissue outside of the lymphatic system.

FAB classification
French–American–British classification of leukemias by morphological means.

Fluconazole
A drug effective in the treatment of fungal infections; also known as Diflucan.

Fludarabine
A drug effective in chronic lymphocytic leukemia; it is also used in high doses as conditioning treatment for reduced-intensity stem cell transplant; also known as Fludara.

Fluorescence *in situ* hybridization (FISH)
This is a technique which evolved from the combination of molecular cloning and hybridization. Specific fluorescently tagged DNA probes are used to visualize small genetic changes, as well as to map the chromosomal locations of genes.

Follicular lymphomas
The second most common form of lymphomas. They are characterized by their indolent clinical behavior.

G-CSF
See granulocyte colony-stimulating factor (below).

Ganciclovir
An anti-viral drug used to treat cytomegalovirus infections.

Gemtuzumab oganomycin
A monoclonal antibody linked to the microbialtoxin calicheamycin which is effective in the treatment of acute myeloid leukemia; also known as Mylotarg or GO.

Gene
The basic unit of heredity. It is one of many short sequences of DNA that contains the information to make a specific protein.

Gene-expression (microarray) profiling
Gene-expression profiling is a genomics technique that enables simultaneous screening of tumors to express tens of thousands of genes at a time; this creates a molecular profile of the RNA in the tumor sample in a semi-quantitative fashion.

Gene therapy
The replacement of defective or missing genes or the addition of useful genes by means of genetic engineering.

Genetic engineering
The technology which allows researchers to pluck genes from the chromosomes, or to insert genes.

Genetics
The study of inherited traits or characteristics.

Genomics
The study of the structure and composition of the material encoding these genetic instructions.

Genotype
Inherited genes; in general these genes remain unchanged during the individual's lifetime, unless they are subjected to a spontaneous mutation (rarely).

GM-CSF
See granulocyte–macrophage colony-stimulating factor (below).

Graft-versus-host disease (GvHD)
An adverse reaction to recipient tissues resulting from attacking immunologically different donor T lymphocytes. It is usually seen after an allogeneic stem cell transplant, but can rarely occur following a blood transfusion.

Graft-versus-tumor effect (GvT)
A beneficial reaction whereby donor T lymphocytes attack recipient cancer cells.

Granisetron
A drug that prevents or reduces nausea and vomiting associated with chemotherapy; also known as Kytril.

Granulocyte
A type of leukocyte that ingests and destroys foreign bodies; also known as neutrophil.

Granulocyte colony-stimulating factor (G-CSF)
An hemopoietic growth factor which stimulates the production of neutrophils (granulocytes).

Granulocyte–macrophage colony-stimulating factor (GM-CSF)
An hematopoietic growth factor which stimulates the production of both the neutrophils (granulocytes) and monocytes (macrophages).

Guthrie blood spot card
The Guthrie card, invented by Robert Guthrie in 1959, is about the size of a playing card and is like blotting paper. The mother's name (not the baby's) is recorded together with the date of collection. The card has four spots of dried blood. A drop of blood is usually collected from the baby by a heel prick and placed on the Guthrie card. The cards are regarded as a health record and stored for up to 50 years. They serve an important role in the screening of many genetic disorders.

Hematologist
A physician (doctor) who specializes in the treatment of blood diseases.

Hematopoiesis
See hemopoiesis (below).

Hemopoietic growth factors (HGF)
A family of biological agents which are useful in the treatment of hematological cancers.

Hemopoietic stem cell (HSC)
Hemopoietic stem cells, also referred to as simply 'stem cells', are the primitive cells in the bone marrow which have the potential to self-renew and differentiate into cells of all hemopoietic lineages: red blood cells, white blood cells and platelets.

Hemopoiesis
The process of blood cell development and differentiation; also known as hematopoiesis.

Hemostasis
The process whereby bleeding (hemorrhage) following an injury (vascular) is arrested.

Hair cell leukemia
A rare form of chronic lymphocytic leukemia characterized by the appearance of peculiar leukemia cells with long cytoplasmic villi resembling hair.

Haplotype
A haplotype is a group of closely linked alleles that tend to be inherited together. They can be used to map human disease genes accurately.

Helicobacter pylori
A bacterium which is causally associated with gastric lymphomas.

Hickman catheter
A central venous catheter often used in the treatment of patients with hematological cancers.

High-dose treatment
Chemotherapy used at five or more times the conventional dose to overcome potential drug resistance in residual disease. It is sometimes combined with total body irradiation (TBI). This treatment's objective is to be myeloablative and the patient will require support with a stem cell transplant.

HLA
The acronym for human leukocyte antigens, see below.

Hodgkin lymphoma
A form of lymphoma, first described by Thomas Hodgkin; also known as Hodgkin's disease.

Human leukocyte antigens (HLA)
The major factors determining compatibility between stem cell donors and recipients.

Human T-cell lymphotropic virus (HTLV)
A virus implicated in certain kinds of leukemias.

Humoral immunity
The part of the immune system that protects the individual from infection by the actions of mature B lymphocytes (plasma cells) which are responsible for antibody production.

Hydroxyurea
A drug used to treat chronic myeloid leukemia and related disorders; also known as Hydrea.

Hyperdiploidy
Leukemic cells, usually ALL cells, with more than 50 chromosomes. This is often a relatively good prognostic feature.

Idarubicin
A drug similar to daunorubicin, but with fewer adverse side-effects and, possibly, more efficacious in the treatment of acute myeloid leukemia; also known as Idamycin.

Imatinib
A novel drug which inhibits the oncoprotein thought to be the principal cause of chronic myeloid leukemia; also known as Glivec or Gleevec.

Immune deficiency
Inadequacy in the body's natural protective mechanisms.

Immunosuppression
The process of 'damping down' the body's immune system to prevent graft rejection in stem cell transplant recipients. During this period the immune system does not function adequately and makes the individual highly susceptible to infections.

Induction treatment
Initial therapy designed to eliminate all evidence of leukemia and restore normal hemopoiesis; also known as remission induction.

Interferon alfa (IFN-α)
A biological molecule (cytokine) which is useful in the treatment of diverse types of cancers, particularly chronic myeloid leukemia and myeloma.

Interleukin
A biological molecule (cytokine) which can be useful in the treatment of certain cancers, particularly kidney cancer, and also in the treatment of some hematological cancers.

Juvenile myelomonocytic leukemia (jMML)
A very rare form of chronic leukemia usually found in children under the age of 5 years; it actually bears very little resemblance to chronic myeloid leukemia.

Keratinocyte growth factor (KGF)
A cytokine which helps in the prevention and treatment of mucositis (inflammation and ulcers of the mouth); also known as Palifermin.

Large granular lymphocytic (LGL) leukemia
An unusual lymphoma which arises from 'natural killer' lymphocytes.

Lenalidomide
A new drug, related to thalidomide, which appears to be effective in the treatment of MDS associated with 5q- and multiple myeloma; also known as Revlimid.

Lenograstim
A form of G-CSF (see above).

Leukemia
Leukemias are a group of cancer disorders characterized by the excessive accumulation of abnormal white cells in the bone marrow and peripheral blood; literally 'white blood'.

Leukocytes
The white blood cells responsible for combating infection and destroying alien material.

Leukapheresis
See apheresis (above).

Lymphoblastic lymphoma
A cancer of the precursor cells of T and B lymphocytes.

Lymphocytes
Types of leukocytes that may secrete substances to destroy invading organisms. See B lymphocytes and T lymphocytes.

Lymphoma
Lymphomas are a heterogeneous group of cancers that originate in lymphoid cells in lymph nodes or other lymphoid tissue.

Magnetic resonance imaging (MRI)
Magnetic resonance imaging is a fundamentally different method of obtaining images from CT. It relies on a powerful static magnetic field and the various properties of the protons (hydrogen ions) in the different tissues. When a strong magnetic field is subjected to certain radio waves of a specific frequency (radiofrequency), the protons will resonate at an exact frequency that depends on the field strength of the magnet. The radio signal emitted back by the protons when the radiofrequency is switched off can be detected in a receiver coil and a detailed image built up.

Maintenance therapy
Treatment which is offered following the successful elimination of cancer cells; better described as continuation treatment; also known as post-remission therapy.

Major histocompatibility complex (MHC)
The specific set of genes that determine an individual's HLA status.

Mantle cell lymphoma
A unique indolent variety of lymphoma which resembles other indolent lymphomas morphologically, but has a specific (BCL-1) oncogene.

Megakaryocyte
Large cells (multinucleated) in the bone marrow from which platelets are produced.

Melphalan
A drug which is effective in the treatment of myelomas; in high doses it is often used as a conditioning treatment for stem cell transplants; also known as Alkeran.

6-Mercaptopurine (6MP)
A drug used in acute lymphoblastic leukemia maintenance treatment.

Metastasis
The passage of malignant cells around the body from the site of origin to establish the same cancer elsewhere.

Methotrexate
A drug which is effective in the treatments of leukemias, lymphomas and many other forms of cancer; it is also effective in the prevention of GvHD.

Mitozantrone
A drug like daunorubicin but with fewer side-effects; also known as mitoxantrone or Novantrone.

Molecular remission
The complete disappearance of a specific molecular marker, for example BCR/ABL gene, as assessed by a validated molecular technique.

Monoclonal antibody therapy
Antibodies which are targeted against a specific antigen on a cancer cell and can lead to immunological cell killing.

Monoclonal gammopathy of undetermined significance (MGUS)
A condition where a patient is noted by chance to have a paraprotein in the blood but no other features to suggest myeloma.

Monocyte
A type of leukocyte which helps fight infections.

Mucosa-associated lymphoid-tissue (MALT) lymphoma
An indolent extranodal lymphoma usually associated with specific cytogenetic abnormalities, such as trisomy 13. In the stomach, it can be associated with infection by a bacterium called *Helicobacter pylori* (see above).

Mycophenolate mofetil (MMF)
An immunosuppressive drug which is effective in the treatment of GvHD.

Mycosis fungoides
An indolent skin (cutaneous) T-cell lymphoma.

Myeloablation
The killing of bone marrow cells by chemotherapy and/or radiotherapy. The term usually refers to the complete or near-complete destruction of the bone marrow.

Myelodysplastic syndromes (MDS)
Disorders characterized by ineffective hemopoiesis (see above) leading to bone marrow failure and a high probability of malignant transformation to acute myeloid leukemia.

Myeloma
Multiple myeloma (typically referred to as simply myeloma) is a cancer which arises from the plasma cells (B lymphocytes) in the bone marrow and is characterized by the production of an abnormal protein called a paraprotein.

Mutation
An alteration in the DNA sequence of a gene.

Neulasta
A long-acting form of G-CSF; also known as pegfilgrastim (see above).

Neupogen
A form of G-CSF; also known as filgrastim (see above).

Neutrophil
A type of leukocyte; also known as a granulocyte (see above) and a polymorph. It is the most mature form of leukocyte.

Non-Hodgkin lymphoma
A form of lymphoma; also known as non-Hodgkin's lymphoma.

Ommaya reservoir
A small implantable port which is connected to a catheter placed in the brain (ventricle) and can be used for the administration of intrathecal chemotherapy (see below).

Oncogene
A cancer-causing gene.

Oncologist
A physician (doctor) specializing in the treatment of cancers; also known as a medical oncologist.

Ondansetron
A drug that prevents or reduces nausea and vomiting associated with chemotherapy; also known as Zofran.

Pamidronate
A drug which is effective in the treatment of bone disease associated with myelomas; it is also effective in the treatment of high blood calcium levels; also known as Aredia.

Palfermin
See Keratinocyte growth factor (KGF).

Pancytopenia
A reduction in all cellular elements of the blood (red blood cells, white blood cells and platelets) to below normal levels.

Pentostatin
A drug which is effective therapy for hairy cell and chronic lymphocytic leukemias; it is also useful in the treatment of low-grade lymphomas; also known as Nipent.

Performance status
A globally understood assessment of a patient's functional ability. A popular scale is that introduced by Karnofsky, which ranges from 0% (dead) to 100% (totally free of any symptoms).

Peripheral blood stem cell transplant
See stem cell transplant.

Peripheral T-cell lymphoma
A type of high-grade lymphoma.

Phenotype
The physical or other effect of the genotype.

Philadelphia chromosome
An abnormal chromosome 22 in the leukemic cells of most patients with chronic myeloid leukemia.

Plasma cell leukemia
A type of leukemia characterized by the presence of more than 20% plasma cells in the peripheral blood.

Plasmacytoma
A localized collection of monoclonal plasma cells.

Platelets
Blood cells which are produced from megakaryocytes (see above) and are required for the prompt arrest of a bleed (hemorrhage) following an injury to a blood vessel; see hemostasis (above); also known as thrombocytes.

POEMS syndrome
A rare syndrome, associated with myelomas and related cancers, in which a blood paraprotein (M) is associated with a peripheral nerve problem (polyneuropathy – P), organ enlargement (O), hormonal disturbances (called endocrinopathy – E) and skin darkening (S).

Positron emission tomography (PET) scan
An imaging technique that depends on the metabolic activity of abnormal areas which are then projected as a metabolic image and may be more sensitive than conventional anatomical imaging, such as a computed tomographic (CT) scan.

Prednisone
A steroid which is often used as part of combination chemotherapy for the treatment of hematological cancers.

Primary amyloidosis
A condition in which tissue deposition of amyloid, a fibrillary protein material derived from plasma cell proliferation, occurs.

Primary cerebral lymphoma
An aggressive type of lymphoma arising from the central nervous system.

Primary tumor
The mass of cells (a tumor) which is at the original site of a cancer.

Prolymphocytic leukemia (PLL)
A variant of chronic lymphocytic leukemia, which can either arise *de novo* or as a consequence of chronic lymphocytic leukemia transforming.

Prophylaxis
Prevention of a disease or complication of therapy.

Proto-oncogene
Normal genes which when 'activated' by various mechanisms lead to a disturbed growth pattern which can in turn lead to a malignant growth. They are made up of sequences of DNA which are susceptible to mutation.

Purging techniques
Methods by which tumor cells are selectively removed from the stem cells harvested from the bone marrow or peripheral blood.

Radiotherapist
A physician (doctor) who specializes in the treatment of cancers with radiotherapy (radiation therapy); also known as a radiation oncologist or a clinical oncologist.

Radiotherapy
This is a form of intensive treatment used to kill cancer cells by interfering with their growth; it is also known as radiation therapy.

Rasburicase
Rasburicase (Elitek; Fasturtec) is a recombinant form of the enzyme urate oxidase, which is an effective treatment for high uric acid levels. This drug is useful in the treatment of the tumor lysis syndrome.

Red blood cells
See erythrocytes (above).

Reduced-intensity allogeneic stem cell transplant
A stem cell transplant between individuals where the conditioning treatment (preparatory regimens) is not myeloablative, as is the case in a conventional allogeneic stem cell transplant; also known as non-myeloablative or mini-transplants.

Relapse
Recurrence of a disease following remission.

Remission
The period during which there is no evidence of disease.

Retrovirus
A virus which may be involved in causing some types of cancer.

Reverse barrier nursing
Nursing techniques designed to protect a patient from infection.

Rituximab
A monoclonal antibody which is effective in the treatment of lymphomas; also known as Rituxan or Mabthera. It may also be useful in some non-cancerous conditions, such as rheumatoid arthritis.

RNA
Ribonucleic acid is a messenger substance which carries genetic information within a cell.

Sanctuary sites
Areas of the body which are difficult for anti-cancer drugs to reach.

Sargramostim
A form of GM-CSF (see above); also known as Leukine.

Second cancers
Second cancers are new cancers which arise as a rare complication of treatment given for a previous cancer.

Sézary syndrome
The 'leukemic' phase of mycosis fungoides, an indolent skin (cutaneous) T-cell lymphoma. It is characterized by the presence of circulating atypical T lymphocytes.

Sirolimus
An immunosuppressive drug which is effective in the treatment of GvHD; also known as rapamycin.

Skeletal survey
Radiographs of the axial skeleton usually carried out in patients with myelomas.

Small lymphocytic lymphoma
This is the tissue manifestation of chronic lymphocytic leukemia (see above).

Spinal fluid
The fluid surrounding the brain and spinal cord.

Spinal tap
A procedure in which a needle is inserted in the space between the lining (meninges) of the spinal cord. It is used to administer chemotherapy treatment (called intrathecal therapy) in patients with acute leukemias at high risk of the central nervous system being involved with disease.

Stem cell
See hemopoietic stem cells above.

Stem cell transplant (SCT)
A transplant using hemopoietic stem cells. When stem cells are derived from the bone marrow, the transplant is referred to as a bone marrow transplant; when the source of stem cells is peripheral blood, it is referred to as a peripheral blood stem cell transplant.

Supportive therapy
Treatment to counter the adverse effects of cancer therapy and to otherwise support the patient.

Syngeneic stem cell transplant
A stem cell transplant between identical twins.

T lymphocytes
Lymphocytes which are produced in the thymus gland and mature in the bone marrow. They provide humoral immunity.

Tacrolimus
A drug which is effective in the treatment of GvHD; also known as FK506.

Thalidomide
A novel drug which works by depriving cancer cells of their blood supply and is effective in the treatment of myelomas and graft-versus-host disease; also known as Thalomid.

6-Thioguanine
A drug which is sometimes used in the treatment of acute myeloid leukemia.

Thrombocyte
See platelets (above).

Thrombocytopenia
A reduction in the total number of platelets.

Thrombopoietin (TPO)
An hemopoietic growth factor which stimulates the production of megakaryocytes and platelets; also known as Neumega.

Tissue typing
The process of finding a suitable stem cell donor for a particular patient.

Topoisomerase enzymes
Topoisomerases are a group of powerful enzymes involved in the coiling and uncoiling of the DNA molecules. Topoisomerase I inhibitors are drugs like topotecan; topoisomerase II inhibitors include anthracyclines such as daunorubicin, and epidophyllotoxins such as etoposide.

Total body irradiation (TBI)
Total body irradiation is sometimes used in conjunction with high-dose chemotherapy and stem cell transplantation.

Total parenteral nutrition (TPN)
Nutrition given intravenously because a patient cannot feed normally.

Tumor
Literally a swelling, but commonly used to mean a mass of cancer cells.

Tumor lysis syndrome (TLS)
A condition which is usually due to the rapid destruction (lysis) of cancer cells by the treatment, resulting in vast quantities of cellular material which overwhelms the filtration systems in the kidneys.

Tumor suppressor gene
A gene that acts to prevent cell growth. If a mutation occurs in this gene, the individual becomes prone to developing a cancer.

Umbilical cord stem cell transplant
An allogeneic stem cell transplant carried out by the use of umbilical cord-derived stem cells.

Vinblastine
A drug, which is effective in the treatment of hematological cancers, particularly Hodgkin lymphoma.

Vincristine
A drug often used in the treatment of lymphoid cancers and myelomas.

Voriconizole
An anti-viral drug which is effective in the treatment of serious fungal infections; also known as Vfend.

Waldenström's macroglobulinemia
A type of myeloma in which a high concentration of immunoglobulin M paraprotein is found.

White blood cells
A synonym for leukocytes.

Zoledronic acid
A drug which is effective in the treatment of bone disease associated with myelomas; it is also effective in the treatment of high blood calcium levels; also known as Zometa.

Appendix I

Sources of information and support for patients with leukemias, lymphomas and myelomas

General

Cancer BACUP
3 Bath Place
Rivington Street
London EC2A 3JR, UK
Tel 0208 7613 2121
Website: www.cancerbacup.org.uk

Cancer Care Society
11 The Cornmarket
Romsey, Hampshire SO51 8GB, UK
Tel 01794 830 300
Website: www.cancercaresoc.org.uk

Macmillan Cancer Relief
89 Albert Embankment
London SE1 7UG, UK
Tel 0800 808 2020
Website: www.mackmillan.org.uk

Marie Curie Cancer Care
89 Albert Embankment
London SE1 7UG, UK
Tel 020 7599 7777
Website: www.mariecurie.org.uk

National Cancer Alliance
P O Box 579
Oxford OX4 1LB, UK
Tel 0870 7700 2648
Website: www.nationalcanceralliance.co.uk

USA

American Cancer Society
Patient Services Department
1559 Clifton Road NE
Atlanta GA 30329-4251, USA
Tel 800 227 2345
Website: www.cancer.org

Cancer Care, Inc.
1180 Avenue of the America
2nd floor
New York NY 10036, USA
Tel 800 813 4673
Website: www.cancercareinc.org

National Cancer Institute
Cancer Information Service
9000 Rockville Pike
Bethesda MD 20892, USA
Tel 800 422 6237
Website: www.nci.gov.org

Patient Advocate Foundation
780 Pilot House Drive
Suite 100-C
Newport News VA, USA
Tel 757 873 6668
Website: www.patientadvocate.org

Specialist

UK

Leukaemia Research Fund
43 Great Ormond Street
London WC1N 3JJ, UK
Tel 020 7405 0101
Website: www.lrf.org.uk

Lymphoma Association
P O Box 386
Aylesbury
Buckingham HP20 2GA
Tel 01296 619 400
Website: www.lymphoma.org.uk

International Myeloma Forum-UK
9 Gayfield Square
Edinburgh EH1 3NT
Tel 0800 980 3332
Website: www.myeloma.org.uk

Leukaemia Care Society
2 Shrubbery Avenue
Barbourne
Worcester WR1 1QH
Tel 0800 169 6680
Website: www.leukaemiacare.org.uk

USA

Center for International Blood and Bone Marrow Transplant Research
(CIBMTR),
Health Polity Institute
Medical College of Wisconsin
8701 Watertown Plank Road
P.O. Box 26509
Milwaukee, WI 53226, USA
Tel 414 456 8325
Website: www.ibmtr.org

Cure for Lymphoma Foundation
215 Lexington Avenue
11th floor
New York NY 10016-6023, USA
Tel 212 213 9595
Website: www.cfl.org

Friends of the José Carreras
International Leukemia Foundation
1100 Fairview Avenue North   (D5-100)
P O Box 19024
Seattle, WA 98109, USA
Tel 1 206 667 7108
Website: www.carrerasfoundation.org

International Myeloma Foundation
2120 Stanley Hills Drive
Los Angeles CA 90046, USA
Tel 800 452 2873
Website: www.myeloma.org

Leukemia and Lymphoma Society of America
600 Third Avenue
New York NY 10016, USA
Tel 800 955 4572
Website: www.leukemia-lymphoma.org

Lymphoma Research Foundation of America
8800 Venice Boulevard
Suite 207
Los Angeles CA 90034, USA
Tel 310 204 7040
Website: www.lymphoma.org

Research

UK

Cancer Research UK
National Office
P.O. Box 123
Lincoln's Inn Fields
London WC2A 3PX, USA
Tel 444 207 121 6699
website: www.cancerresearchuk.org

European Group for Blood and Marrow Transplantation
Central Registry Office
Department of Haematology
MacDonald Buchanan Building
Middlesex Hospital
Mortimer Street
London W1N 8AA, UK
Tel 444 207 380 9772
Websie: www.ebmt.org

Blood & Marrow Transplant Newsletter
1985 Spruce Avenue
Highland Park IL 60035, USA
Tel 847 831 1913
Website: www.bmtnews.org

Center for International Blood & Marrow Transplantation
Health Polity Institute
Medical College of Wisconsin
8701 Watertown Plank Road
P.O. Box 26509
Milwaukee, WI 53226, USA
Tel 414 456 8325
Website: www.ibmtr.org

International Myeloma Foundation
2120 Stanley Hills Drive
Los Angeles CA 90046, USA
Tel 800 452 2873
Website: www.myeloma.org

National Cancer Institute
website: nci.nih.gov.org

Other useful global sources

The Cancer Council Australia
GPO Box 4708
Sydney NSW 2001
Tel 02-9036 3100
Website: www.cancer.org.au

Cancer Patients Assistance Society of NSW (CPAS)
Website: www.cancerpatients.com.au

CanTeen
Tel 1800 639 514
Website: www.canteen.com.au

Children's Cancer Institute Australia
Tel 1800 685 686
Website: www.ccia.org.au

Myeloma Foundation of Australia
P O Box 2014
Mt Waverley
Vic 3149
Tel 03 9807 9841
Website: www.myeloma.org.au

Canada

Bikers Memorial Cancer Fund
Tel 1 902 497 9005
Website: www.bikersmemorialfund.tripod.com

Canadian Cancer Society
National Office
Suite 200
10 Alcorn Avenue
Toronto, Ontario M4V 3B1
Tel 1 416 961 7223
Website: www.cancer.ab.ca

Candlefighters Cancer Foundation
55 Eglinton Avenue East, Suite 401
Toronto, Ontario M4P 1G8
Tel 1 416 489 6440
Website: www.candlelighters.ca

Denmark

Foreningen Kræftens Bekæmpelse
Strandboulevarden 49
2100 København Ø
Tel 35 25 75 00
Website: www.cancer.dk

Eire/Ireland

BMT Support
Bone Marrow & Stem Cell Transplant Support Group
Tel 1 800 200 700
Website: www.bmtsupport.ie

Irish Cancer Society
43/45 Northumberland Road
Dublin 4
Tel 01 2310 500
Website: www.irishcancer.ie

France

CNP Assurances
4 place Raoul Dautry
75716 Paris Cedex 15
Tel 01 4218 8888
Website: www.cnp.fr

Fondation Croix saint Simon
125 rue d'Avron
75020 Paris
Tel 01 44 64 43 53
Website: www.cdrnfxb.org

Société Française D'Accompagnement et de Soins Palliatifs
106, Avenue Emile Zola
75015 Paris
Tel 01 45 75 43 86
Website: www.sfap.org

Germany

Bundesorganisation
Selbsthife Krebs e.V.
Campus-Virchow Klinikum
Augustenburger
Platz 1
13353 Berlin
Tel 030 450 578 306
Website: www.selbsthilfekrebs.de

Deutsche José Carreras Leukämie
Stiftung, e.V.
Arcistrasse 61
80801 München
Tel 089 272 9040
Website: www.jcarreras.com

Holland/the Netherlands

Dutch Cancer Society
KWF Kankerbestrijding
P O Box 75508
1070 AM Amsterdam
Tel 020 570 05 00
Website: www.kwfkankerbestrijding.nl

Vereniging 'Ouders, Kinderen en Kanker' (VOKK)
Schouwstede 2d
NL-3431 JB Nieuwegein
Tel 030 2422 944
Website: www.vokk.nl

Hong Kong

Children's Cancer Foundation
Room 702, Tung Ning Building
125 Connaught Road Central
Hong Kong
Tel 852 2815 2525
Website: www.ccf.org.hk

Iceland

Icelandic Cancer Society
P O Box 5420
IS 125 Reykjavik
Tel 354 540 1900
Website: ww.krabb.is

India

Cancer Patients Aid Association
Website: www.cpaaindia.org

Italy

Federazione Cure Palliative
G. Salvini Ospedale
Viale Forlanini 121
Milano
Tel 02 9902 2062
Website: www.fedcp.it

La lega Italiana Per la Lotta
Contro I tumori
Sede Centrale
Via A. Torlonia 15
00161 Roma
Tel 06 442 5971
Website: www.legatumori.it

Norway

Kreftforeningen
Postboks 4 Sentrum
0101 Oslo
Tel 22 86 66 00
Website: www.kreftforeningen.no

Romania

Pavel
Sos. Mihai Bravu 311-313
Bl. SB1, Sc 1, Ap., 1
Sector 3
Bucuresti
Romania
Tel 021 344 2885
Website: www.asociatiapavel.home.ro

Singapore

Children's Cancer Foundation
KK Women's & Children's Hospital
100 Bukit Timah Road, Level 7
Singapore 229899
Tel 6297 0203
Website: www.ccf.org.sg

Spain

Asociación Española contra el cancer
C/ Amador de los Rios 5
28010 Madrid
Tel 031 941 38
Website: www.todocancer.com

Fundación Internacional José Carreras
Muntaner 383 2n
08021 Barcelona
Tel +34 93 201 0588
Website: www.f.carreras.bcn.servicom.es

Sweden

Cancerfonden
David Bagares gata 5
101 55 Stockholm
Tel 08 677 1000
Website: www.cancerfonden.se

Switzerland

Fondation José Carreras Pour La Lutte
Contre La Leucemie
Case Postale 85
CH 1217 Meyrin 2
Website: www.jcarreras.com

La Chrysalide
Centre de soins palliatifs La Chrysalide
Rue de la Paix 99
23012 La Chaux-de-Fonds
Tel 032 913 35 23
Website: www.chrysalide.ch

Lega Svizzera Contro il Cancro
Website: www.swisscancer.ch

Appendix II

General references and suggested further reading

General

Cancer: The Evolutionary Legacy by Mel Greaves, Oxford University Press, 2002.
Oxford Textbook of Oncology; ed. Souhami, Tannock, Hohenberger and Horiot; 2nd edition, Oxford University Press, 2001.

Leukemias

Acute Leukaemias, Mughal and Goldman, in *Textbook of Cancer*, ed. Price and Sikora, Arnold Press, 5th edition 2002; 6th edition (planned).
Chronic Leukaemias, Mughal and Goldman, in *Oxford Textbook of Medicine*, Oxford University Press, 2003.

Lymphomas

Lymphomas, Armitage, in *Oxford Textbook of Medicine*, Oxford University Press, 2003.

Myelomas

Multiple Myeloma, Kyle and Rajkumar. *N Engl J Med* 351: 1860–73, 2004.

Index